Bircher-Benner Manuals

Manual for patients with hypertension, cardiovascular disease and arteriosclerosis

Dietary instructions
for prevention and healing,
with recipes,
detailed advice
and a treatment plan
from a medical centre
for state-of-the-art healing

Dr. med. Andres Bircher
and colleagues of the
Bircher-Benner Medical Centre
Lilli Bircher, Pascal Bircher and
Anne-Cécile Bircher

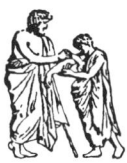

EDITION BIRCHER-BENNER
CH-8784 BRAUNWALD

Bircher-Benner manuals

1. Manual for patients with multiple sclerosis and degenerative nervous diseases
2. Manual for patients with liver and gallbladder conditions
3. Manual for families and children
4. Manual of fresh juices, raw vegetables and fruit dishes
5. Manual for improvement of the immune system and against susceptibility to infection
6. Manual for mountaineers and athletes
7. Manual for diabetics
8. Manual for support and preventive therapy for lung diseases
9. Enjoy food without table salt
10. Manual for patients with rheumatism and arthritis
11. Manual for men with prostate conditions
12. Manual for patients with kidney and bladder conditions
13. Manual for venous diseases
14. Manual for patients with gastrointestinal conditions
15. Manual for nutrition during pregnancy and lactation
16. Manual for gynaecological problems and menopause
17. Manual for the prevention of cancer and accompanying therapies
18. Manual for headache and migraine
19. Manual for patients with hypertension, cardiovascular disease and arteriosclerosis
20. Manual for overcoming anxiety and depression
21. Manual for patients with skin diseases or sensitive skin
22. Manual for persons suffering from stress
23. Manual for persons suffering from allergies
24. Manual for prevention of dementia and Alzheimer's disease
25. Manual for internal treatment of eye problems
26. Manual for treatment of weight problems, overweight, and anorexia

These manuals are the results of global research, the development of the medical art and science across more than a century and the experience of the renowned Bircher-Benner Klinik. The reader will feel the helpful support of the well-informed physician at every step of the way.

17th edition fully revised 2015. Translated from the original German

All rights reserved, including the right of reproduction in excerpts, photomechanical reproduction or translation
info@bircher-benner.com   www.bircher-benner.com

Book orders: edition@bircher-benner.com
© Copyright Edition Bircher-Benner, CH 8784 Braunwald
® The trademarks Bircher and Bircher-Benner are protected worldwide
Printed in Germany

The suggestions in this book have been carefully reviewed by the authors and the publisher. However, we cannot assume any guarantee.
The autors and the publishers hereby disclaim all liability for personal injury, property damage and all types of financial loss.

Cover design: Kösel Media GmbH, Krugzell
Overall production: Kösel, Krugzell

Table of Contents

Preface to the 17th edition 9

Introduction 10

The healthy heart, an astounding organ 13
    The heart and its functions 13
    The systemic circulation 14
    The pulmonary circulation 15
    The capillaries and the basic substance of the soft connective tissue 15
    Degeneration and regeneration, and the obsolescence of calorie calculation . . 16

Arteriosclerosis, a widespread disease 18
    The risk factors for cardiovascular diseases 18
    The problem of small amounts of alcohol 19
    Oxidative stress, an important contributing cause 20
    What precisely is arteriosclerosis and how does it develop? 21
    The importance of fat metabolism, obesity and cholesterol 23

The importance of fatty acids 26
    Saturated fatty acids 26
    Unsaturated fatty acids 26
    Monounsaturated fatty acids 26
    Polyunsaturated fatty acids 27
    The pharmacological effect of the omega-6 and omega-3 fatty acids 27
    The suitable ratio between polyunsaturated fatty acids 28
    The risk of oxidation of highly unsaturated oils 29
    The problem of vegetable margarines, cream and butter 29

The importance of cholesterol 30
    The cholesterol metabolism 30

The effect of nutrition on the cholesterol levels in the blood	31
Cholesterol metabolism disorder and gallstones	32
Cholesterol and coronary heart disease	32

The importance of proteins and amyloidosis 37

The importance of carbohydrates and sugar for arteriosclerosis 38

The importance of vegetarian nutrition in the prevention of coronary heart disease 40
- The effect of almonds and nuts on arteriosclerosis 40
- The effect of fruits and vegetables on arteriosclerosis 40

The antioxidative effect of vegetarian raw food, the importance of secondary plant substances 41
- The importance of wholemeal cereals 42

Bircher-Benner's healing diet and order therapy 43

Hypertension 45
- Blood pressure regulation 48
- Pulmonary hypertension 50
- Treatment of hypertension with medication 51

Angina pectoris 54
- Stable angina pectoris 54
- Unstable angina pectoris 54
- Prevention and treatment of heart attack 55

Heart attack 56
- The risk factors for heart attack 57
- Caring for a heart attack victim 75
- Complications of heart attack 75
- Prevention of heart attack 58

Cardiac insufficiency or chronic heart failure 59
- Dietary treatment of cardiac insufficiency 60

Heart valve defects 61
- Mitral valve stenosis 61
- Mitral insufficiency 62

Aortal valve stenosis	63
Aortic insufficiency	64
Pulmonary valve stenosis	64
Pulmonary valve insufficiency	64
Tricuspid valve stenosis	65
Tricuspid valve insufficiency	65
Inflammatory diseases of the heart	66
Myocarditis	66
Toxic myocardial damage	66
Autoimmune inflammation of the heart	66
The symptoms of myocarditis, treatment and prognosis	66
Endocarditis	67
Aneurysm	68
Aneurysm dissecans of the aorta	68
Aneurysms of the cerebral arteries	68
Stroke (apoplexy)	69
Renal artery stenosis	71
Carotid artery stenosis	72
Peripheral vascular disease (PVD)	73
Arrhythmia	74
Supraventricular extrasystoles	74
Ventricular extrasystoles	75
Atrial flutter and atrial fibrillation (absolute arrhythmia)	75
Tachycardia	77
Inflammation of the arteries	79
Vasculitis	79
Regulative treatments of naturopathic healing for cardiovascular patients	82
Climate therapy and terrain treatments	82
Hydrotherapy	82

Classical homoeopathic treatment	83
The new scientific acupuncture	84
Neural therapy	85
General directives for the treatment and prevention of arteriosclerosis and cardiovascular diseases	86
The healing regime	88
Secondary plant substances	94
Menu	96
Menus for various raw food regimes	96
1. Fresh Juice Fasting (bed/juice day)	96
2. Full Juice Day	96
3. Fruit Fasting Days	97
4. Raw Vegetable Menus (for stage-II diet)	98
Daily menu	98
The Recipes	100
Fruit Juices	100
Vegetable Juices	100
Potato Juice	101
Gruel to Accompany Juices	101
Birchermuesli	101
Sprouted cereal grains	103
Linomel muesli according to Dr. Johanna Budwig	103
Raw vegetables and salads	103
Salad dressings	104
Table for Choosing Suitable Salad Dressings	108
Milk Types	109
Plant fats, oils and butter	109
Gentle cooking and steaming/sautéing	110
Soups	110
Vegetables	113
Salads of cooked vegetables	118
Potato dishes	118

Cereal Dishes	122
Sauces	124
Sandwiches	126
Desserts	127
Table for Raw Food Diet	130
Healthful teas	131
Recipes	133
Notes	134
Index	142

Preface to the 17th edition

This manual is based on wide experience in the treatment of patients who suffered from cardiovascular diseases and, where still possible, were healed by Bircher-Benner's order therapy. Former editions have been supplemented with many references and insights from clinical, epidemiological and fundamental research. The dietetic section has also been slightly revised, without sacrificing the high quality of Bircher's recipes. For people who are willing to take the early signs and risk factors of cardiovascular disease seriously, and who wish to know how to prevent the disease from developing in order to avoid severe disability or death from heart attack or stroke, this book provides indispensable information and practical instruction.

Since its establishment by Dr. Maximilian Oscar Bircher-Benner, the order therapy and its healing effects for cardiovascular diseases have been observed carefully for more than a hundred years at the Bircher-Benner clinic and in private practices. Throughout those years, the thousands of patients who succeeded in stopping the progression of their diseases were our greatest teachers. With a strong will to be healed, they successfully followed the instructions of the order therapy and enabled great insights to be made which are only now emerging in general medical research. Our experience that hypertension can be reversed by diet, and that arteriosclerosis can be reversed (even in coronary vessels) by long-term and careful application of our diet, has been proven scientifically and without objection for approximately two decades.

For a transition to a more healthful lifestyle, nutrition is of vital importance. It leads to regeneration of the large regulation systems, a new opening towards the outer world and the inner self which permits the healing forces of the organism, body and soul to begin their work. To quote a section of Bircher-Benner's book *Vom Werden des neuen Arztes* (Becoming a Physician for the Future): 'The wonders of the soul remain closed to those who continually ignore the laws of nutrition. Power and depth of inner experiences depend on nutrition–this is the actual meaning of nutrition. Taking care of one's body and nutrition is senseless unless a new development and awakening of inner powers result from it.'

The entire order of life plays an important role, especially with regard to circulatory disorders. True healing is not possible without a basic deepening of knowledge about the sense of life, the orders of life, as well as the relationship to work, society, oneself and the people with whom we share our lives. The beginning of this path is the great question of responsibility towards others and oneself. It is a path that is well worth taking.

For the treating physician, this book is a great help in the instruction and support of his patients.

Dr. med. Andres Bircher

Introduction

Anyone suddenly beset by a cardiovascular disease will feel threatened at his very core. After all, the cardiovascular system plays a vital role in our existence. Blood pressure may be low for years, then suddenly complaints begin and blood pressure rises, usually after sustained psychological stress (e.g. anger or permanent stress at work). The loss of regulation is manifested in vertigo, headaches, preoccupation, inner unrest and anxiety. After a brief examination performed to rule out rare causes, the general practitioner prescribes the first medication, noting that it will be required *ad vitam* and must be taken regularly to prevent dangerous consequences. Medication to reduce blood pressure often acts quickly. The patient grows accustomed to taking the medication regularly and begins to become calmer. However, the disease will continue to progress silently. The dose must be increased, and new medicines are added with both desired effects and side effects. But where is the question about the cause? None of the thousands of respondents we asked really knew. Therefore the path went from the first symptoms directly to medication, without eliminating the causes. This deficit is not due to the absence of good will, but rather is an expression of a general misunderstanding between the current paradigm of medical science and human biology. Usually the medical diagnosis is a straightforward description of symptoms and does not deal with the cause. The path usually goes directly from diagnosis to pharmacotherapy, without exploring the cause of the disease and without treating its origins. This deficit in medical action and thinking must be remedied, because it has pernicious consequences.

In spite of tremendous medical efforts, statistics of the World Health Organisation reflect a continuous increase of cardiovascular diseases in all more or less industrialised countries. The technical and pharmacological progress in angiology and cardiology has been remarkable and has led to indubitable improvement in the life expectancy of persons suffering from cardiovascular diseases. In the USA, life expectancy has increased by 26 % over the past 10 years, while fatalities have declined by 12.9 %.[1]

However, it has become evident that these encouraging results are countered by a steady increase in the number of affected persons, and that the prevention previously recommended does not work because it only addresses a very small part of the causes. Treatment often comes too late, and is limited more or less to dealing with the consequences and complications. Too often, the specialist's medical history resembles an impressive life-extending patchwork of surgical and angiological treatments, as in the insertion of stents into narrowed vessels, vein grafts, the mechanical occlusion of the left atrial appendage, insertion of artificial heart valves, carefully designed pharmacotherapy and even heart transplants. The genius of pharmacological research has brought forth several valuable medicines that we would not want to do without in the advanced stages of cardiovascular disease. However, it is in these late stages specifically that treatment of the cause is of vital importance, since the disease will continue to progress despite considerable medical efforts.

In 2006, the number of people in the USA who suffered from one or several cardiovascular diseases was estimated to be 81.1 million. Furthermore, 73.6 million Americans suffered from high blood pressure and 17.6 million from coronary heart disease, while 8.5 million suffered a heart attack in 2006 and 8.5 million Americans died from the consequences of a cardiovascular disease in the same year.[1]

Arteriosclerosis begins early. Chosen at random, three hundred young fallen soldiers (21.1 years old on average) of the Korean War were examined. Autopsies revealed that 77.3 % of these soldiers had already showed massive arteriosclerotic changes of the coronary vessels.[2] Because of unsuitable nutrition, even young children are suffering from heart problems as a result of manifest arteriosclerosis.[3,4,5,6,7] Angiologists speak of an 'iceberg phenomenon', since 85 % of the arteriosclerotic changes go unnoticed for a long time. Arteriosclerosis can be healed if no sensitive structures such as heart valves or important regulation centres have been affected. In the medical centre founded by Maximilian Bircher-Benner in Zurich in 1897, the progress of scientific research, practical experience and treatment was continually observed and integrated. At the centre, several decades' experience in treatment not only diminishes this disease by means of medication and surgery, but may even heal it. Even at the later stages, progression of the disease can be stopped. Patients intelligent enough to consistently address the causes, which lie in the poor nutrition and unnatural lifestyles commonly found today, have the best chances for complete healing, provided that the disease has not yet (or only just) manifested itself. They will not only overcome the already-present arteriosclerotic changes, but will be rewarded with a general improvement of the quality of their lives and their resilience. Even in a late stage of the disease, patients who make changes in accordance with the instructions in this book will be rewarded. Patients can expect clear improvement of the condition and renewed mental and physical strength.

The human organism is equipped with such an extraordinary plethora of free reserves, regulation, compensation and emergency solution options that keeping disease in check and unnoticed for many years is an invaluable gift of nature. However, we should not wait to change our lifestyle and nutrition habits until those regulation mechanisms fail and the disease leaves irreversible damage. Medication, including homoeopathy, can help in a crisis and relieve suffering, but it can never heal the disease. Surgical and angiological interventions can save lives, but they will leave behind weaknesses which the disease will relentlessly attack. True healing of arteriosclerosis is only possible by consistent treatment of the cause. We refer to this path as 'order therapy'. Nutrition and lifestyle must be adjusted precisely to biologically specified conditions. Nutrition must have a very high ordering of energy potential, which contains the regenerative information of sunlight that enters all living beings through photosynthesis. Like breast milk, nutrition must be 'ecologically' composed, without any stress on the metabolism due to nonsensical excess. Nutrition must contain a very high share of essential nutrients and vital substances, and be free of all irritants such as coffee, alcohol, industrially spoiled ready-made meals, and appetite and flavour enhancers. Nutrition must also be free of roasted substances, alcohol and other drugs that give us the illusion of stimulation while actually only weakening and paralysing our life force. We yearn for such stimulants again and again, in the hope of reducing this paralysis, if only temporarily.

We need to relearn how to harmonize with the life rhythms of nature, with which all of our regulation mechanism and hormone cycles are aligned. All of this will increase our life force and inner harmony and soon free us to order our relationships and our working world. Those who do not want to stop at the common treatment of symptoms but who strive for healing from arteriosclerosis and hypertension will find all the necessary information in this book, as well as practical instructions. The experienced physician will find this book a great help in the consultation and support of his patients. This treatment will become a fascinating exploration, a trusting act of cooperation between doctor and patient.

The healthy heart, an astounding organ

The heart and its functions

More than any other organ, the heart symbolises life. Like the ticking of a clock, its metronomic beating structures the course of the years and reminds us of our mortality. A strong heart is not only a symbol of love, joy and suffering, but also of life itself. The heart's performance never ceases to amaze us. It exceeds that of engines produced by man. The heart runs day and night without interruption or maintenance for 80 years, and without cleaning, repair or replacement. It beats about 100,000 times per day, 40 million times per year and has the pumping capacity of almost three billion heart pulsations over a period of 70 years. It pumps seven litres of blood per minute (300 per hour) through a vascular system approx. 100,000 km in length, or one-and-a-half times the circumference of the equator.[8]

This is the resting capacity of the heart, and every stimulus affecting the body requires increased performance by the heart. How much must this irreplaceable motor of life have been abused to finally fail! And yet the number of patients with cardiovascular diseases continues to increase and does so at both ends of the age spectrum, starting at increasingly young ages.

The heart can never rest as most other muscular organs do and must continue to pump even during sleep. At least all vital functions are switched to protection mode and are able to rest at night, sparing the heart sudden performance demands. The heart does get a little rest during sleep, when most organs are dormant. Blood pressure is lower during sleep than at any other time, while the need for circulation in other body areas is reduced. The coronary vessels are relieved, and all processes of life (except those that serve recovery) are dampened and adjusted to greatest economy.

The heart consists of a hollow muscle that is approximately fist-sized, internally structured into four independent compartments by two large separating walls in length and width: two atria and two ventricles. The ventricles are lined with hard tissue, and the inner layer of the heart the (endocardium) has a strong connective tissue layer covered by a thin membrane the (endothelium). The entire heart muscle moves in a heart sac the (pericardium) in which it can perform its pumping motions, sliding smoothly while embedded in a small quantity of fluid. The right atrium receives the venae cavae coming from the entire body and pumps the blood into the right ventricle through a valve with three flaps the (tricuspid valve). This in turn pumps the blood into the pulmonary arteries with every beat of the heart. The valve that separates the ventricle from the atrium closes like a pump valve, followed by the pulmonary valve, so that no blood can flow back into the right ventricle. It is surprising how the flaps of the tricuspid valve, attached only at the edge and limited in movement by stretched chord-like tendons *(chordae tendineae),* are able to resist this enormous pressure. At further passage through the capillaries of the lungs, the blood emits carbon dioxide to the alveoli and saturates the red blood pigment (haemoglobin) with oxygen, turning it a bright red. The pulmonary veins take the bright blood to the left atrium. This will contract while the ventricles relax, pumping it through the mitral valve into the left ventricle of the heart. Together with the right heart, the left heart contracts while occluding the mitral valve between the left atrium and the left ventricle, to pump the oxygen-enriched blood into the aorta and from there into the large systemic circulation. The aortic valve closes at once so that no blood can flow back into the left ventricle. The pumping action of the ventricles is called the systole; the relaxation phase of the ventricles, during which the atria fill them, is called the diastole.

Heart muscle fibres have the property of electrically discharging themselves rhythmically and consequently contracting. Special fibre bundles dominate self-discharge by discharging faster than the remaining muscle (Purkinje fibres). In the right atrium lies the pacemaker centre, the sinus node. In a healthy heart, the sinus node produces the fastest frequency and conducts the stimulus through conductive fibres of the atrium down to the second pacemaker centre, the Aschoff-Tamara node, which on its own would produce a slower frequency of just under 40 beats per minute. From there, the stimulus conduction fibres continue into the ventricles in two finely branched bundles, which on their own would discharge even more slowly. The dominant effect therefore is top to bottom, with the faster frequency dominating the slower one.

On the one hand, the vegetative nervous system regulates the heart frequency by sympathetic fibres coming from the ganglia of the sympathetic trunk of the 5th thoracic vertebral segment. In the event of stress, general excitement, joy or anger, they increase the heart frequency via the sinus node (positive dromotropic effect) and increase the output power of the heart (positive inotropic effect). At general relaxation, the parasympathetic nerve fibres of the heart reduce the heart frequency and thus the output power (e.g. in sleep). With these two antagonists, the sympathetic nervous system and the parasympathetic nervous system, the vegetative nervous system controls the heart, similar to the way a carter reins in his horse.

The systemic circulation

The large aorta divides into two arm arteries (arteria subclavia) as well as two outer and two inner head arteries (arteria carotis externa and interna). The outer carotid artery supplies the face and the outer head organs, while the inner one supplies the brain. Another artery for the brain rises up the spine to the back of the head, where it is connected to the front artery. The downwards aorta branches off into the arteries for the liver (arteria hepatica), the spleen (arteria lienalis) and the kidneys (arteria renalis); other branches go to the stomach, the pancreas and the intestine (Truncus coeliacus, arteria mesenterica superior and inferior). These three branches supply the intestine with oxygen-enriched blood. In the capillary network of the intestinal mucosa, the nutrients, bacterium toxins, gall acids and fats enter the blood after becoming transportable by being packed into tiny transport bubbles (chylomicrons). The intestinal veins are called portal veins, since they combine again and carry the blood from the intestine to the liver portal and from there through new branches to the individual liver lobules. In the pelvic area, the aorta splits into an inner and an outer pelvic artery; the inner one supplies the pelvic organs (bladder, uterus, prostate) and the outer one the legs. The arteries continue to branch down to the smallest arterioles that regulate the blood flow to the capillaries with their tiny muscles.

The pulmonary circulation

The right atrium takes up the blood from the larger vena cava of the systemic circulation and pumps it into the right ventricle through the tricuspid valve at low pressure during the relaxation phase of the ventricles. The strong contraction of the ventricle closes the flaps of the tricuspid valve very tightly, preventing blood from returning into the atrium and ejecting it completely into the pulmonary artery. The pulmonary valve also closes at once and prevents the blood from returning into the right ventricle. Like a tree, the pulmonary artery branches very finely down to the lung capillaries. These are embedded in soft connective tissue (matrix), between the soft walls of the alveoli. This is where the gas exchange takes place, in which the dark, venous blood passes the carbon dioxide from the metabolism into the breathing air while taking up oxygen from the breathing air in the blood cells. This turns the blood a bright red.

The inner diameter of the capillaries is only four-thousandths of a millimetre, while the size of the red disc-shaped dented blood cells is seven-thousandths of a millimetre. The wisdom of creation requires the blood cells to roll up into a wedge shape to pass through the narrow capillaries. In this process of rolling up, the blood cells take up a multiple of the oxygen from the breathing air that they can if ill, when they have lost this ability because their membranes have been damaged by a metabolism overloaded by senselessly supplied nutrients.[9] Capillary microscopy at the nail bed permits a direct and vivid observation of this phenomenon.

The capillaries and the basic substance of the soft connective tissue

The branching of the smallest vessels into the capillaries in the large systemic circulation is infinite.

The basic regulation in the matrix of the soft connective tissue is as follows:

All body tissues are shot through with soft connective tissue (matrix). All cells of all organs, the muscle and connective tissue fibres, and the blood capillaries are embedded in the soft connective tissue. This matrix is filled with a molecular network of sugar protein molecules (proteoglycans). Even the small channels in the bone, the spaces between the columns of the liver cells in the liver lobules, the dentine and the fine pores of the tooth enamel are penetrated by this molecular network.
There is no direct connection between blood capillaries and the cells. The nerve fibres also end blindly in this network of the basic substance[10] of the soft connective tissue and do not touch the cells directly anywhere. Any substance that is to be taken from the blood to the cells must pass this molecular network of the basic substance. Thus it acts as a molecular screen. The protein share of the sugar protein molecules of this network stabilises it and the sugar molecules form the bristles, as if two brushes were being pushed against each other. Only electromagnetic powers (Van der Waals' forces) bind them together. In this way, the sugar molecules can shift continually. It has been proven that the network of the proteoglycans in the basic substance of the soft connective tissue is an ideal medium for conducting and storing information as we understand it from computer science.[10]

Any information that must get from the nerve endings to the cells or from the cells to the nervous system is conducted through this network of proteoglycans. In fact, every stimulus started anywhere in the body is routed into the entire body through this network.[10] Thus this molecular network of the basic substance of the soft connective tissue stores the information of our biological system: the information of life. Each of the roughly 15 trillion cells of our bodies transfers its own information to our vegetative nervous system through the basic regulation system, and from there all the way to our awareness through the large centres of the brain stem. The information of all cells that we are made up of is our feeling of life and our subconscious and conscious memory.

Degeneration and regeneration, and the obsolescence of calorie calculation

Physicists are aware of two types of energy: orderly and chaotic. Orderly energy saves information. Chaotic energy cannot save anything. Heat energy is chaotic energy. Sunlight is the most highly ordered energy. Its information is similar to a large symphony. Listening to a symphony does not produce heat, but it provides information: a highly orderly sound structure that triggers precise sensations and feelings. With its complex oscillations, sunlight conveys and orders the genetically specified information that is needed for growth, differentiation and the regeneration of all life on earth.

One green leaf contains about one million chlorophyll funnels. At the base of each funnel, there are two chlorophyll α molecules. The funnel reflects the incoming light into the base, where the chlorophyll α molecules enter into maximum resonance, synchronised with the oscillations of the solar radiation (coherence). They convert the energy from this resonance into UV light, which makes them light up (invisibly to our eyes). This light flows through the entire plant body all the way into the tips of the roots.[14]

All living cells store UV light in their molecules, and particularly in the ring-shaped molecules. The double helix of the genetic material in the cell cores stores by far the most light. The double helix (DNA) can coil to the right or left and can form protrusions shaped like clover leaves, radiating specific UV light spectrums.[11] The double helix of the DNA serves as a cavity resonator for the rhythmic laser-amplification of UV light in our cells.[12] For a laser to take up work, it must receive a certain amount of energy. Bio-physicians call this minimum energy supply the laser threshold. In their experiments, researchers of the international academy for biophoton research measured the laser threshold in plant tissues.[11]

Just like plants, human and animal cells store UV light in their DNA.[13, 14] However, we lack the ability to photosynthesise, and direct application of sunlight to the skin is not nearly enough to keep our laser-light storage above the laser threshold.

The plant's cell stores the photons from sunlight in extremely large amounts. It could be shown that ultra-weak cell radiation is nothing but a kind of leakage radiation, a tiny leak of the UV-light through the cell membrane. Measurements have shown that laser amplification of the light is ten^{10} times stronger in the DNA than that provided by technical laser devices.[11] The inside of the cells thus represents an incredible light space.

Our photon storage must be fed daily by a sufficient amount of living photon-containing foods (fresh fruit and vegetables).[15, 16, 17, 18]
The transmission of the information contained in the cellular UV light of the living foods from photosynthesis to our

organism takes place by coherence. This means that our own sensation of life, our life energy and life information, is repeatedly renewed and reordered in the roughly 15 trillion cells of our body by entering into a shared resonance with the oscillation patterns of sunlight upon transfer of the photons.

If fresh living foods are missing from our nutrition, the photon content in our cells will decline. The light content will decrease until it falls below the laser threshold. The cells partially revert from the principle of order the (the coherence principle of Prigogine) to the chaos principle of thermodynamics, and then degenerate.

We consider disease a loss of order, a loss of ordered information. The programme of life enters into disorder and the lack of living nutrition makes reordering impossible. Many experiments conducted at the University of Novosibirsk and elsewhere[18] show that the complex processes of biochemistry in our cells are controlled by information. If there is a lack of living nutrition, this information will no longer be continually renewed and ordered. Consequently, the complex biochemical processes of our cells will be thrown into disarray. This is why Fresh raw fruit and vegetable food is important for its energy: it renews and strengthens the ordering resonance.

Arteriosclerosis, a widespread disease

There has been considerable research and publication about the manner and the creation of degenerations of the arterial walls that lead to arteriosclerosis. Genetics alone cannot explain the immense increase of the disease over the past decades. Stress (i.e. in this case a fast, unfulfilled life full of friction, or whatever the inappropriate constant stress may consist of) can only take its full effect due to 'stress conditioning factors', as Selye, the founder of the stress theory, has shown. These factors are found in nutrition, lack of movement and sleep, toxins scattered from infection foci, bad air, smoking, pollution, increasingly massive electro smog from the pulsated high-frequency radiation of wireless telephony and electrical devices. These can have a large and sometimes triggering effect. The basic item remains indisputably nutrition. What bears the main fault with regard to nutrition, however, is still subject to debate: fat (quantity and quality), cholesterol content, refined carbohydrates or excess protein (quantity and type).

If you have followed these questions for decades, you will have found recently – and not without a certain relief – that clarification is on the horizon. One can now say that arteriosclerosis results from an oversupply of food and stimulants, food with a concentrated nutrient content but a lack of auxiliary substances (vital substances), more or less desaturated from industrial processing, 'enriched' with chemical additives and impaired in their correlations.

In spite of all efforts, the statistics have shown a massive increase of this disease since World War II, with all its disastrous consequences that arrive increasingly early in life. To examine arteriosclerosis, researchers at the University of Texas performed 1,160 autopsies on infants, children and teens, aged between neonates and adults 29 years of age. Fully 45 % of the infants at the age of 8 months already showed fatty streaks and foam cells (macrophages filled with oxidised cholesterol) in places that are particularly exposed to blood flow. By puberty the numbers increased, and at the age of 12–14, the muscle layers of the arterial walls were also shot through with fatty deposits. Of these young people, 8 % already had arteriosclerotic atheromes (plaques) in the intracellular substance.[19] In New England, the risk factors in 204 children and young adults (ranging from 2 to 39 years old) who had died in accidents were analysed. Further studies showed that arteriosclerosis is increasingly becoming a paediatric problem.[20, 21, 22, 23, 24] In 2003, the American Cardiology Association (ACA) issued a statement on this problem. Causes cited were poor nutrition with obesity and diabetes type II, which had increased alarmingly among children.[25]

The risk factors for cardiovascular diseases

It took almost 100 years before smoking was recognised as a high risk factor. Other recognised risk factors are hypertension, diabetes, a family history of heart attacks, obesity, sedentary lifestyles, nutritional fat-metabolism disorders with high LDL cholesterol and triglyceride levels (or the rare congenital hyperlipidaemias), stress at work and anger. Forty percent of all heart attacks occur in the early morning hours, between 6 a.m. and 10 a.m., and particularly on Mondays. Heart attacks are also due to emotions (e.g. during football world championships).[26] Scientific studies on the influence of anxiety, depression, social isolation and chronic stress lead to contradictory results.[27, 28] Other risk factors are a lack of vitamin D or migraines with aura.[29] People with blood type A are slightly more at risk.

The frequency of arteriosclerosis is difficult to record statistically. It is called an iceberg phenomenon, since only approx. one-tenth of the occurrences of the disease become evident with the first symptoms which lead people to see a doctor. Until then, many people live in apparent health in the symptom-free stage of the disease, when the organism is still able to circumvent the problem. This was the case in the children and teenagers, and the Korean soldiers.[2] The disastrous consequential diseases of arteriosclerosis, heart attack and stroke (apoplexy), by contrast, have been proven statistically. In 2003, 10.9 % of all deaths in Germany were due to coronary heart disease, and 7.5 % were due to heart attack. In 2012, 5.2 % of all deaths in Germany were due to heart failure (cardiac insufficiency). In the USA today, cardiovascular diseases are the most common cause of death, even ahead of accidents and cancer.

The frequency of heart attack is based on lifestyle and nutrition. In Japan, 1 out of 1000 persons suffers a heart attack each year; in Switzerland and France, 2 out of 1000; in Germany and Austria, 3 out of 1000; in Scandinavia, 4 out of 1000; and in England and Hungary, 5 out of 1000. According to the statistics of the German Federal Office, 52,000 persons died of a heart attack in 2011. Socially disadvantaged persons are more at risk and do worse during the first year after a heart attack than persons from the privileged classes.[30] Since 2000, the frequency of heart attack in Germany has fallen slightly, from 67,000 to 52,000 cases.[31]

The most tragic complication of arteriosclerosis is stroke. In Germany, 4 out of 1000 persons each year suffer a stroke from occlusion of a brain artery (apoplexy) or from a haemorrhage in the brain. Bleeding into the brain fluid (subarachnoid haemorrhage) is rare (6 out of 100,000 persons). Strokes are the third most common cause of death in Germany.

The problem of small amounts of alcohol

The harm of 'small' daily amounts of alcohol is currently disputed. Studies of the University of Bordeaux have shown that people with low wine consumption[32] (approx. 2 small glasses of wine/day = approx. 30 g of pure alcohol/day) are a little less likely to die of the consequences of coronary heart disease than abstinent persons or persons who drink larger quantities of alcohol. The vast publicity of this result is understandable, since it lends credence to a daily habit. Wine-growing areas in particular saw a general recommendation from many doctors to their patients to drink red wine every day. In countries such as France, where wine is drunk regularly, the connection between coronary heart disease and blood fats (cholesterol) can be documented much less clearly. This is called the 'French paradox'. However, even relatively low amounts of alcohol (42 g of pure alcohol/day) increase the cholesterol level considerably.[21] It is noteworthy that people who drink 'a little' wine with a meal usually take in much more than 30 g of pure alcohol/day. A Japanese prospective study over seven years showed that background characteristics (risk factors) such as smoking, nutrition, etc. of the "moderate drinkers" in the French study must have been much better than those of the abstinent persons and those who had consumed more alcohol.[33] In a carefully considered editorial in the *Journal of the American Medical Association,* the problem is dealt with in more detail.[34] A table lists all persons who are harmed even by the smallest amounts of alcohol: people with a family history of alcoholism, pregnant women, and people suffering from diseases of the liver, the pancreas, weakness of the heart, excessive blood triglyceride values, degenerative nervous diseases and certain blood diseases. In this study even the 'smallest amounts' of alcohol are considered harmful, amounts which should be completely avoided before work or driving. In fact, increased risk with machines and vehicles and reduced mental performance have been documented in numerous cases.[35, 36, 37, 38] In light of the fact that nowadays people drive cars or operate machines almost every day, the recommendation of 'small amounts of alcohol' becomes problematic indeed.

In 1992, Wannametzee et al. from the Royal Free Hospital in London documented in a large number of patients that persons suffering from angina pectoris are much more likely to die of sudden heart failure than abstinent persons if they drink even very small amounts of alcohol.[39]

Alcohol leads to oxygen deficit in the liver cells, which will promote fatty degeneration of the liver lobules even with a low daily amount. Alcohol is the cause of chronic pancreatitis. Medical science notes that regular consumption of 16 g of pure alcohol per day is dangerous to the pancreas. This corresponds to 4 dl of beer, 1.1 dl of red wine, 4.5 dl of cider or 50 ml of brandy or spirits. A digestif taken regularly will cause precipitation (sludge) to form in the fine pancreatic ducts. The sludge produces chronic inflammation of the pancreas. Alcohol also damages the glandular cells directly and impairs the function of the sphincter of the excretory duct of the pancreas, causing the digestive enzymes activated in the small intestine to flow back and provoking self-digestion of the pancreas. In Germany, 8000 persons (70 % of them men) are hospitalised every year because of chronic pancreatitis. Pancreatic cancer results from the chronic inflammation of the pancreas. Regular consumption of alcohol, even in small amounts, is the indisputable cause of this.[40] This fact illustrates the scope of the problem caused by the recommendation made under the influence of the 'French paradox'.

Oxidative stress, an important contributing cause

Unsuitable nutrition, irritants, environmental stress, disorderly lifestyle, ionising, electromagnetic and UV-A radiation all cause the organism to suffer from oxidative stress. This creates a metabolic environment in which the amount of reactive oxygen compounds (R.O.S., or reactive oxygen species) exceeding the physiological limit is created.

These highly reactive oxidising substances are molecules with at least one unsaturated electron pair, conditions which make them especially reactive. They are produced in the mitochondria, the 'power plants' of the cells that break down glucose through electron transfer and the enzyme Cytochrome P 450-oxidase. This produces the super oxide anion radical O_2-hydrogen peroxide (H_2O_2) and the hydroxide radical (OH) or nitroxygen (NO).

Healthy cells can neutralise these highly reactive oxygen compound with neutralising substances that they keep at hand. The most important antioxidative substance provided by the body is glutathione, a peptide that it produces from the three amino acids: glutamine acid, cysteine and glycine. Other important antioxidants are ubiquinone (of coenzyme Q 10), vitamins A, C and E, selenium and many secondary plant substances.

Oxidative stress occurs in the metabolism when these reserves have been depleted. Oxidised glutathione can no longer be sufficiently returned to its active, reduced form, since the enzyme glutathione reductase is depleted, as well as other detoxication enzymes such as peroxide dismutase and catalase. The highly reactive oxidants (R.O.S.) thus remain in the metabolism, where they can damage large molecules (macro molecules) inside and outside the cells. This has dangerous consequences. The unsaturated fatty acids of the cell membranes are oxidised (lipid peroxidation), which causes the destruction of the mitochondria and also requires the cells to expend considerable energy to maintain their electrical membrane potentials. Additionally, there will be damage to proteins (protein peroxidation) and the hereditary material (DNA-peroxidation), damage which causes the DNA-molecules of the hereditary material to split (genetic mutations) and may lead to the conversion of healthy cells into tumour or cancer cells. This is a premature ageing process, which considerably impairs life expectancy.[41, 42, 43]

Glucose metabolism (in the respiratory chain of the mitochondria) produces water as the end product. In about 2 % of all cases, errors happen (e.g. an oxygen atom will connect to one instead of two hydrogen atoms). This will always create a highly reactive fission product of water: the hydroxide radical (OH^*). This free radical is highly reactive because the oxygen atom of the OH radical is looking for an additional electron from any other molecule with great force. Other radicals include nitrous oxide (NO^*), the chloride radical (CL^*) and the bromide radical (Br^*).

The importance of the free radicals is currently subject to great scientific interest in connection with researching the causes of various neurodegenerative diseases, such as Alzheimer's disease, amyotrophic lateral sclerosis (ALS), Chorea Huntington and Parkinson's disease. Many studies suggest destruction of the brain stem ganglions by free radicals as a cause of these increasingly common diseases. Diabetic neuropathy may also be caused by nerves damaged by free radicals.[44]

What precisely is arteriosclerosis and how does it develop?

Arteriosclerosis means hardening and narrowing in arteries. It is a degenerative systemic disease that leads to a focal-scarred reconstruction process in the middle (Tunica media) and inner (Intima) layers of the arterial walls, including deposits of collagen, oxidised, degenerative blood fats and proteins (amyloids), blood clots (thrombi), cholesterol and calcium crystals. Capillary microscopy enables the experienced doctor to identify this disease in the very early stages. The innermost third of the arterial walls is supplied with oxygen and nutrients directly from the blood flowing inside. The outer two thirds, however, are a complex organ. Muscle and connective tissue layers are tightly overlaid to absorb the enormous stress from the continuous heart beats. To feed these two thirds, supply them with oxygen and remove the metabolism waste products from them, the arterial walls, like other organs, are supplied by smaller arteries (vaso vasorum) that lead into them and form a dense capillary network between the connective tissue and muscle layers that are embedded in the basic substance of the soft connective tissue (matrix), with its dense network of proteoglycans between all the cell and fibre layers.

As early as the 1930s, using capillary microscopy it was possible to demonstrate on living persons that 1) unsuitable nutrition with less than two-thirds fresh raw fruit and vegetable food would cause the capillary loops to expand and grow heavier, making them wind like meandering rivers and leak; and 2) that inflammation forms around them because of deposits of degenerative proteins and fats (amyloides).[45] This pericapillary inflammation is due to the deposit of metabolic slags in the molecular network of the proteoglycans in the basic substance of the soft connective tissue, slags from nutrients senselessly supplied in a surplus that the metabolism is unable to handle. At the same time, it can be seen that the red blood corpuscles have lost their ability to roll up, and have to squeeze painstakingly through the narrow capillaries. This considerably reduces oxygen supply to the cellular tissues. These degenerative changes, with the deposit of amyloides in the molecular proteoglycan network of the soft connective tissue, occur not only at the arterial walls but in all tissues and organs. They mark the beginning of all degenerative diseases.

The changes in the arteries start particularly where there is a strong blood flow that injures the innermost cell layer, the vascular endothelium. In the early years of life, the first superficial deposits of degenerative (oxidised) fats are found there, particularly in the form of oxidised low-density cholesterol (LDL). This change is reversible. If the oxidative stress and inadequate nutrition continue, the deposits will condense into larger inflammatory foci. These will swell. Immune cells will recognise the oxidised lipids as degenerative material and distribute interleukin monocytes, a special type of white blood cell that turns into macrophages (scavenger cells) to remove the slags. Like amoebae, they wander into the arterial wall and ingest the degenerative material in many tiny bubbles to dissolve it. The excess of oxidised lipids from the blood makes this a Sisyphean task. More and more foam cells filled with degenerative fats and amyloid will thus be deposited in the inflammatory foci of the arterial wall, especially the middle layer.

These foci will swell and increasingly block up the inner space of the vessels. The narrow areas in the coronary vessels produce chest pains because of a lack of oxygen during effort, stress or anger (angina pectoris). If the arteriosclerotic plaques break up inwards, blood clots will form to occlude the vessel. These may also be transported elsewhere. In a coronary vessel, this means a heart attack. Since there is no bypass circulation, an entire patch of heart muscle wall will die. In a brain artery, this will cause a stroke (apoplexy), which will cause another (smaller or larger) part of the brain to die instantly. Such infarctions are possible in the organ arteries as well, e.g. in an intestinal artery (mesenterial infarction); or, more rarely, a renal or spleen artery; or, more frequently, a leg artery, which will cause disabling, cramp-like pain after the patient has walked a certain distance. The pain recedes once the patient stops (claudicatio intermittens). At the aorta or in strongly pulsating brain arteries, such arteriosclerosis foci may also break up outwards. First, the pulsations soften the vessel outwards (aneurysm) before breaking open towards the brain (haemorrhagic insult) or the meninges (subarachnoid haemorrhage), which will cause severe disability, paralyses or immediate death. The aortal wall may be split open on the inside with widespread arteriosclerosis (aneurysm dissecans) and will sooner or later break open outwards (aneurysm rupture), a deterioration which is always fatal. All of these are tragic events and create extreme conditions of suffering, danger and fear as potentially disastrous consequences of arteriosclerosis.

The importance of fat metabolism, obesity and cholesterol

With the knowledge of molecular-biological basics regarding storage of excess nutrients in the basic substance of the soft connective tissue, and thus the relocation of the transit route between the cells and their surrounding structures,[10] we can understand that widespread poor diet and frequent adiposity result in a massive impairment (nutrition and metabolism) of the tissues and the liver.

The adipose person is actually in a constant condition of hunger, a vicious circle in which he eats because he is hungry, but which provokes the opposite conditiwithons: further stress on the liver and clogging of the basic substance, with even worse cellular metabolism deficits. After all, the adipose person not only eats too much; he also eats the wrong things.

It has become clear that adiposity can be treated sustainably and successfully not by calorie reduction, but by raw juice treatment and subsequent raw food therapy for nine months with unrestricted food consumption.[46] In the vicious circle of adiposity, intestinal symbiosis (the impaired intestinal flora), with the related weakening of the liver and the enterohepatic cycle, is also important.[46] There is little being done in adiposity research at the present time. At all events, a 10 % sustainable weight reduction could be achieved with a basic order-therapeutic treatment and a supporting change of lifestyle, and the doctors then observed a significant improvement in the blood pressure values and serum cholesterol. A fibre addition to the common hypocalorific diet alone reduced cravings and eliminated constipation.[47]

The liver is the key organ for regulating the fat and cholesterol levels in the blood. These levels express the metabolisms of the liver. There are many studies on reduction of the cholesterol level by means of dietetic measures.[48, 49] They are of great interest to the medical profession because of heart attack risk. In 1988 in the USA, the NCEP (National Cholesterol Education Program) was published, after many studies had documented the advantage of lipid reduction to counter heart attack risk. Results from the extensive Coronary Primary Prevention Trial had asserted the famous 2:1 relation, according to which a cholesterol reduction by 1 % reduces coronary heart disease risk by 2 %. The dietary provisions of the AHA (American Heart Association) were adjusted to these studies.[50]
The Helsinki heart study demonstrated that additional increase of the HDL (high-density lipoprotein) cholesterol values improves this result. Fibres such as bran or psyllium seeds have also been shown to reduce lipids several times.[49, 51, 52, 53, 54, 55]

A positive effect of unsaturated fatty acids (omega-3 fatty acids) has been documented in several studies.[56] It was shown that omega-3 fatty acids improved blood viscosity by helping the red blood cells regain their flexibility.[57] In cases of nephrosis (nephrotic syndrome: protein loss in the urine due to basal membrane damage at the kidneys' capillary loops) there is a strong increase of blood fats as an expression of the regulation disorder of the entire hepatic metabolism.[57]

It was also shown that the serum cholesterol in such patients could be reduced by a drastic reduction of protein in their diet.[58]

Looking at the individual effects separately shows that they all suggest a vegetarian diet. There is a large number of papers which document that vegetable nutrition with a marked reduction of animal products is very effective in reducing lipids.[59, 60, 61] The Heidelberg vegetarian study examined the differences in the overall lipid status of 62 female and 40 male vegetarians, in comparison with a control group of omnivores. Unsaturated oleic acids in particular were taken up more by the vegetarians. The fatty acid composition of the cholesterol esters, triglycerides, free fatty acids and phosphatidylcholin was analysed. In all of these fractions, the fatty acid profile reflected the dietetic lipid intake. Palmitol, vaccenyl-docosahexoaenyl acid remained much looser in the serum of vegetarians. The greatest difference was measured for linoleic acid in all lipid classes, particularly in di- and triglycerides.[62]

These insights were new at the time. When used consistently for therapy, they had a drastic effect on the risk of dying from coronary heart disease by improving the liver metabolism. A drastic reduction of LDL cholesterol and overall cholesterol in the diet reduced the cases of coronary heart disease by 35 % and the need for surgical intervention in the coronary vessels by two-thirds. The 'Coronary Drug Project' and the 'Multiple Risk Factor Intervention Trial', two large-scale prospective studies, documented the long-term effect of lipid reduction. Two other large studies proved the effect of dietetic lipid reduction angiographically as well by contrast sketching of the coronary arteries (CLAS: Cholesterol-Lowering Atherosclerosis Study and FATS: Familial Atherosclerosis Treatment Study). The FATS study additionally showed that an existing condition of arteriosclerosis of the coronary arteries can partially remit under a consistent lipid-reducing diet.[63] In all of these positive results, it must be considered that a drastic dietetic lipid reduction is only possible with very marked limitation of animal food, so that studies cannot only refer to cholesterol. It was shown that the effect of dietetic lipid reduction on coronary heart risk can be clearly improved by regular physical training in overweight men and women.[64]

A breakthrough was achieved by a prospective, randomised control study managed by Professor Ornish at the University of San Francisco, examining the influence of nutrition and 'life style on coronary sclerosis', published in the renowned journal, *The Lancet* in 1990.[65] Over a 12 month period, 28 patients with strong coronary sclerosis were at least partially treated with order therapy. They had a strictly vegetarian diet with a very low share of saturated fats, and they did not smoke. They also received relaxation training and instructions for adjusted physical training. Lipid-reducing medication (statins) was not administered. The control group comprised 20 patients comparable in age, gender and coronary angiography findings (narrowing of the vascular cross section by 40 %). The control group was treated according to all common the recommendations of the American Heart Association, including medication with statins. After one year, another angiography was performed. The order therapy group showed a clear reduction of complaints and expansion of the vessel cross section, from 40 % to 37.8 % (re-opening of the coronary arteries), while the control group had suffered further constriction (on average from 42.7 to 46.1 %) with a clear increase in complaints.

This outstanding work provides an impressive demonstration of the great importance of nutrition for liver metabolism and thus the blood lipid profile and its direct, strong influence on arteriosclerosis. It bears out the decades-long experience of the Bircher-Benner clinic, according to which a suitable change of diet will clear the tissues and permit already-narrowed vessels to open again. In 1995,[66, 67] Dougall et al. also reported on the rapid reduction of the cholesterol level from a low fat, strictly vegetarian regime.

The fatty degeneration of the liver (fatty liver) is often connected to general obesity and hypertension, and frequently with type II diabetes. This symptom complex is called the metabolic syndrome.

Adventist youths (vegetarians) are much less adipose than omnivorous comparison groups.[68]

Vegetarians have only half the mortality risk for any food-dependent chronic diseases, in particular cancer and cardiovascular diseases.[69] This was proven in Berlin in 1990.[70]

The fatty liver can be improved by alcohol abstinence with weight reduction and physical training.[71, 72, 73] With a suitable diet, even in adipose patients with a fatty liver, gallstones will not appear.[74] Malabsorption from celiac disease often leads to a fatty liver.[75] These and other similar papers clearly demonstrate toxic stress of the liver due to excessive stress on the enterohepatic cycle (poisoning of the liver by toxins from the intestine).

The importance of fatty acids

Natural fatty acids are carbon-hydrogen chains with an even number of carbon atoms and a carboxyl end (HO-C=O). Butyric acid is the shortest one, with five carbon atoms. In a healthy intestinal flora, butyric acid is produced from plant fibres (dietary fibre) by bacteria and is very important for the nutrition of the intestinal mucosa cells.

We know more than 400 fatty acids from plant seeds, but only 12 of them are common. Those that our body cannot produce are called essential fatty acids. They are similar to vitamins, as they need to be taken in via food, and in sufficient amounts. Fats are made up of three fatty acids bound to a glycerine molecule. When fatty acids are allowed to react with a sodium or potassium containing alkaline, soap is the result.

The fatty acids are oxidised in the mitochondria, the power plants of the cells, by coenzyme-A (β-oxidation) in the metabolism. Afterwards they can be broken down in the same manner as glucose. Degradation will produce plenty of energy-rich phosphate (ATP = adenosine triphosphate), which supplies the energy needed for the processes of the chemical reaction chains (like a fuel) in many parts of the metabolism.

Saturated fatty acids

For saturated fatty acids, the carbon chain has no double bonds. They occur in plants and even more so in animal fats.

Unsaturated fatty acids

They occur mainly in fruit and vegetable food. They contain one or several double bonds in their carbon chain, which can be spatially in cis or trans positions (same side or opposite). Natural fatty acids have their double bond in the cis position, which causes a spatial bend in the carbon chain at approx. 30 %. The double bond of essential fatty acids must be at least nine carbon atoms away from the acid end, since otherwise there will be no enzymes to make use of them. For humans only two fatty acids are, strictly speaking, essential: linoleic acid and α-linolenic acid.

Monounsaturated fatty acids

These are rich in olive oil and contain only one double bond in their carbon chain. Polyunsaturated fatty acids contain several (usually two) double bonds.

To determine the position of the double bond in the carbon chain, the carbon atoms are counted from the end of the chain that is not the acid end. It is designated with Ω (omega), because it is the last C atom of the chain. If several double bonds are present, as in the polyunsaturated fatty acids, the double bond that is closest to the omega end will determine the designation. Therefore, we differentiate omega-3 fatty acids and omega-6 fatty acids.

Both saturated and unsaturated fatty acids provide plenty of energy, regulate the immune system, brighten the mood and counter fears. They have very different effects on the metabolism.

Monounsaturated fatty acids (olive oil) act positively against cardiovascular risks. They lower the systolic and diastolic blood pressure, and reduce insulin resistance when there is diabetes (lower HbA1C and the fasting blood sugar level).[76, 77]

A study with 13,600 participants showed that a ratio of many unsaturated fatty acids to few saturated fatty acids reduces the risk of cardiovascular diseases.[78] In the Mediterranean area, the share of monounsaturated oils in the energy supply of people is at 16–23 %. In this sense, an exchange of saturated fatty acids (animal fats) produced by mono- and polyunsaturated fatty acids and carbohydrates, as is common in the Mediterranean, leads to a reduction of the cardiovascular risks.[79]

Polyunsaturated fatty acids

Linoleic acid and α-linolenic acid are the essential omega-3 fatty acids. This means that supplying them in food is absolutely vital. Plants contain almost exclusively linoleic acid and α-linolenic acid where omega-3 fatty acids are concerned: flax seed oil approx. 60 %, walnut oil approx. 13 %, rapeseed oil approx. 9 % and soybean oil approx. 8 %.

Fish contains mostly decosahexaenoic acid (DHA) and eicosapentaenoic acid (EPA): salmon 1.8 %, anchovies 1.7 %, sardines 1.4 %, Atlantic herring in vinegar 1.2 %, mackerel 1 % and white tuna 0.7 %. Long-lived predator fish contain methylmercury, which is highly toxic for the nervous system. This is considered a reason for concern starting at a monthly intake of 114 g of swordfish or 454 g of tuna. Sardine, anchovy, mackerel and salmon are much less toxic. Additionally, antibiotics and growth enhancers are often added to fish farm ponds. We must consider that all oceans are polluted with radioactive isotopes from nuclear tests and nuclear power plant disasters and disposals, which are not at all limited to Japan. Because of the currents, all oceans have been radioactively contaminated. Considerable amounts of radioactive Caesium have also been found in Swiss fresh water lakes. Because of the food chain, the plant toxins condense towards animals. Inspections of fish deliveries for toxin content and radioactivity are not regularly performed. The omega-3 oils of fish-oil capsules are chemically denaturated by esterification and chemical reconversion. For all of these reasons, we can neither recommend eating fish nor fish oil capsules to cover the omega-3 oil demand. Fish are usually baked at much more than 100 °C, usually between 140 and 250 °C. There has been little research on what happens to polyunsaturated fatty acids (decosahexaenoic acid DHA and eicosapentaenoic acid (EPA) at such temperatures. These fatty acids are apparently highly sensitive to long storage and heating, so that a large quantity of vitamin E must be added as an antioxidant when heating them.[80] In analogy with the high sensitivity of the vegetable omega-3 oils to oxidation, it can be expected that the baking and roasting of fish will also produce carcinogenic oxidised oleic acids. This is another reason why eating fish for the supply of omega-3 oils cannot be recommended.[81]

The pharmacological effect of the omega-6 and omega-3 fatty acids

The human body converts omega-3 fatty acids into the biologically effective fatty acids decosahexaenoic acid (DHA) at 6 % and to eicosapentaenoic acid (EPA) at approx. 2 %.[82, 83] The conversion rate depends on the amount of triglycerides and omega-6 fatty acids that are taken in with the food at the same time. The Deutsche Gesellschaft für Ernährung (DGE) currently recommends at least 250 mg of EPA and DHA fatty acids. This demand is covered by at least 5 g of linolenic acid or 9 g of flaxseed oil per day. Since this protects from cancer and modulates the immune response, we recommend taking in at least 30 g of flaxseed oil per day. It can easily be added to the Birchermuesli or to salad dressings or directly by taking one tablespoon three times a day.

Omega-6 fatty acids can promote the creation of arachidonic acid by several conversion steps, and thus stimulate the synthesis of inflammation-promoting prostaglandins. Omega-3 fatty acids, in contrast, dampen this effect and weaken it. Omega-3 fatty acids achieve an immune-modulating effect by calming an overactive immune system so that inflammations, allergies and autoimmune diseases will be weakened, while omega-6 fatty acids increase the inflammatory processes.

An overactivated, exhausted immune system raises the risk of cancer. Omega-3 fatty acids counter cancer. They stimulate the T_h2-tier of production of the T4 helper cells, which counter inflammations. Omega-6 fatty acids, in contrast, stimulate the T_h1-tier of T4 helper cells and thus promote inflammatory reactions. In arteriosclerosis foci, an excess of omega-6 fatty acids promotes the inflammatory processes and thus the progression of the disease, while a large amount of omega-3 fatty acids in nutrition counters the degenerative oxidation and inflammation and thus arteriosclerosis.

Both types of highly unsaturated fatty acids are essential, i.e. absolutely vital. Both are very valuable nutrients that the body cannot produce, but that must be taken in at a suitable ratio. Too high a ratio of omega-6 to omega-3 fatty acids will displace the omega-3 fatty acids from shared enzymes and thus inhibit their effect.

The suitable ratio between polyunsaturated fatty acids

Much research has recently been conducted regarding the ideal ratio between omega-6 and omega-3 fatty acids. Ratios of 1:1 to 1:4, i.e. a much higher share of omega-3 than is common, are ideal for health.[84] The most commonly found poor nutrition, however, corresponds to a ratio of 1:8 to 1:10. Even a ratio of 1:3 reduces the inflammatory processes in rheumatoid arthritis.[85] Asthma bronchiale improves even at a ratio of 5:1, but deteriorates clearly even at a ratio of 10:1.[77] A ratio of 2.5:1 inhibits the growth of intestinal cancer significantly, while a ratio of omega-6 to omega-3 fatty acids at 4:1 no longer produced cancer-inhibiting effects.[77] An excessively high omega-6 to omega-3 ratio in food also promotes the formation of blood clots and thrombosis. In addition, such a ratio generally promotes cramps and inflammation and facilitates cancer.[86]

A plethora of data finally was used to calculate a ratio of omega-6 to omega 3 fatty acids of at least 1:5. This ratio has been recommended by international nutrition specialist groups. We recommend a ratio of at least 1:1. This can easily be achieved by addition of one third flax seed oil to olive oil. If sunflower seed is preferred, more flax seed oil must be added as the former contains only small quantities of omega-3 fatty acids.

The risk of oxidation of highly unsaturated oils

It is very important to note that oils with polyunsaturated fatty acids will oxidise when oxygen is added, during long storage, heating or exposure to light. The oxidised fatty acids are strongly suspected of being carcinogenic. Cold-pressed flaxseed oil in particular must be entirely fresh at all times and should be stored tightly closed in the refrigerator and kept in the dark.

The problem of vegetable margarines, cream and butter

Elaidic acid results when oleic acid is hardened for the production of vegetable margarine from oil. The double bonds are moved from the natural cis position in the trans position, and the trans-fatty acids are carcinogenic. Therefore, the use of margarines with hardened oleic acids is not recommended. By law, hardening must be indicated on the packaging. Nut butter is a healthy, unhardened vegetable fat.

Cow's milk, cream and butter also contain trans-fatty acids, since their rumen organisms contain hydrating enzymes. Because of the content of trans-fatty acids and the high share of saturated fatty acids, we recommend that cream and butter be used very sparingly. They can easily be replaced by olive oil when preparing hot meals.

The importance of cholesterol

Cholesterol is a firm white substance that was found in gallstones as early as the 19th century. Its name actually means 'firm gall'. Cholesterol is a very important substance. It is part of the cytoplasmic membrane present in all cells. Cholesterol increases its stability. Together with certain proteins, it contributes to transporting signal substances through the cytoplasmic membrane (cellular membrane). The body contains approx. 140 g of cholesterol, of which 95 % is in the cells and cytoplasmic membrane.

For transport in the blood and the intracellular substance, cholesterol is bound to fat-protein molecules (lipoproteins). The protein parts make this complex soluble in water. There are different lipoproteins of different physical densities that can be separated from each other by centrifugation or electrophoresis. Accordingly, five types of cholesterol-transporting lipoproteins can be differentiated. The most important ones are HDL (high density lipoprotein) and LDL (low density lipoprotein).

The cholesterol metabolism

Ninety percent of cholesterol is produced by the intestinal mucosa and the liver. In adults, this amounts to 1–2 g/day. Only 10 % is supplied by food of animal origin, and vegetarian food contains no cholesterol. The intestine will take in only 100 to 200 milligrams of cholesterol per day. The cholesterol-producing cells of the liver continually measure the cholesterol level and adjust production to demand.

Cholesterol, a vital substance

The body uses cholesterol to produce the steroid hormones of the adrenal cortex: cortisol and aldosterone, which are vital for regulation of the immune system, controlling inflammation phenomena, the regulation of the blood-sugar level and control of the salt metabolism by the kidneys. By side-chain separation, the body also produces pregnenolon from cholesterol, which plays a role in the production of the various female and male sexual hormones (testosterone, estradiol and progesterone). New cardiac glycosides that the body produces from cholesterol have also been discovered. Their effect is the topic of current research. Seven-dehydrocholesterol, an interim product of cholesterol synthesis, serves as a provitamin for formation of vitamin D under the effect of UV-B-radiation of the sunlight.

Cholesterol is also vital as a raw material for the continuous synthesis of bile acids, such as cholic acid and glycocholic acid. Every day about half a kilogram of cholesterol is excreted into the intestine through the bile acids.

Bile acids are required for resorption of all substances from the intestine that are not water-soluble. Cholesterol is also resorbed by the bile acids. Once in the intestine via the bile ducts, 90 % of the bile acids are resorbed again after their work of resorbing the fats from the lower sections of the intestine. This means that only 10 % (about 50 g/day) of the 500 g cholesterol from the bile acids are actually excreted through the intestine.

Regulation of the cholesterol synthesis

Cholesterol synthesis is regulated via different inhibiting systems. HMG-CoA-reductase, a very important enzyme of cholesterol synthesis, is inhibited if the cholesterol level in the liver is high enough. Various proteins have bonding points that, if occupied, will lead to reduction of the cholesterol-forming enzyme HMG-CoA-reductase, which in turn will reduce production of the cholesterol.

The transport of cholesterol in the blood and the tissues

When the intestinal mucosa takes up cholesterol, it immediately packs it into tiny droplets called chylomicrons. In this packaging, the portal vein system transports the cholesterol to the liver. The liver cells will bind the cholesterol to LDL, VLDL and IDL (LDL cholesterol) after its synthesis or resorption from the portal vein blood. Bound to these lipoproteins, the cholesterol reaches all body tissues from the liver. Once in the capillary networks of the tissues, the cholesterol diffuses through the capillary walls into the soft connective tissue with all other nutrition substances, then through the molecular network of the basic substance to the cell membranes, and finally into the cells.

High-density lipoproteins (HDL) and low-density lipoproteins (LDL)

HDL lipoproteins take up the cholesterol excreted from the cells and return it to the liver.
LDL lipoproteins absorb the cholesterol produced by the liver cells and take it into all body tissues.

LDL cholesterol is often inaccurately called 'bad cholesterol', because a raised LDL cholesterol level at a low HDL cholesterol level is statistically associated with a higher risk of cardiovascular diseases.

In fact, a sufficient LDL cholesterol level is extremely important for the supply of all body cells with cholesterol for the membranes and the metabolism. Cholesterol is very important for differentiation of the brain cells. LDL cholesterol values artificially lowered too far by medication with statins may weaken the memory or even cause memory loss.

The effect of nutrition on the cholesterol levels in the blood

Chemically bound in the lipoproteins to be water-soluble for transport in the blood, cholesterol is also bound to fatty acids which are taken in from food. These can be saturated, monounsaturated or polyunsaturated fatty acids, depending on the food. When a diet is high in polyunsaturated fatty acids, the LDL cholesterol level in the blood has been shown to drop. Eating many saturated fatty acids from animal fats will considerably increase the LDL cholesterol level.

The level of HDL or LDL cholesterol in the blood very much depends on nutrition. Vegetarians and particularly vegans have a lower total cholesterol level, a higher HDL and a lower LDL cholesterol level.[62]

The effect of poor nutrition and oxidative stress on cholesterols

LDL cholesterol is broken down by two independent methods. All cell types of the arteries have LDL receptors including the liver cells. Sixty-five percent of LDL cholesterol is broken down directly in the arterial walls and the liver cells (LDL-receptor path). Under conditions of widespread nutrition and oxidative stress, approx. 15 % of the LDL cholesterol is oxidised. This oxidised (and therefore rancid) cholesterol enters the inner layer (intima) of the arterial walls, where it must be broken down by the macrophages, also called scavenger cells. They have special receptors for rancid cholesterol to recognise it and absorb it (phagocytosis). If this breakdown path (scavenger pathway) is overloaded, an increasing number of macrophages filled with rancid LDL cholesterol (foam cells) remain in the innermost layer of the arterial wall (intima), particularly in artery locations with heavy flow. The pathologist calls these yellowish deposits 'fatty streaks'. If the poor nutrition persists, this fattening reaches into the deeper layers of the arterial walls, then the immune system reacts with inflammation. Now other degenerative lipids and proteins (amyloids) settle into the arterial walls. Finally, these arteriosclerosis foci will calcify or break open. Starting with oxidised LDL cholesterol, arteriosclerosis leads to the disaster of complete destruction of the arterial walls, the occlusion of the leg arteries, heart attack, stroke, dissociating aortic aneurysm or subarachnoid haemorrhage.

The cholesterol level
In middle age (35–65 years old), the average cholesterol level of German patients is at 6.1 mmol/litre (236 mg/100 ml). In some parts of China, where vegan diets are common, levels are at 2.3 mmol/l (94 mg/100 ml). The normal value has been specified at between 1.8 and 4.4 mmol/l (70–170 mg/100 ml). Men under 45 years old have a higher overall cholesterol level, while women have a higher one at a later age.

The HDL/LDL-level ratio is often calculated, since it correlates with the cardiovascular risk even more than the overall cholesterol level does. For women in Germany, the average is 3.9, and for men it is 4.9. The ratio of overall cholesterol /HDL for women is 5.7 and for men 7.0.

Hypercholesterolemia
A low overall cholesterol level clearly reduces the risk of cardiovascular diseases.[87, 88]

There are four types of congenital, genetic hypercholesterolemias with an increased risk of cardiovascular diseases. In part, the LDL receptors are incompletely developed. The autosomal dominant hypercholesterolemia affects about one in every 500 persons. This increases the risk of suffering a heart attack at a young age.[89] Examinations in affected families over the last 200 years show that nutrition and lifestyle had a great influence on the frequency of disease.[90]

Cholesterol metabolism disorder and gallstones

Half of gallstones consist of pure cholesterol, and 80 % are high in cholesterol. They are a consequence of poor nutrition. The risk for developing gallstones increases with body weight.[91] A large study in New Delhi has shown that nutrition with a high share of carbohydrates and saturated (animal) fats will cause gallstones.[92] The gall of obese persons contains cholesterol crystals. The slower the passage through the large intestine, the more likely the gallstones will occur. This change is attributable to the changed resorption of the bile acids in the case of obstipation.[93] For more information, see the Bircher-Benner manual no. 2: *Manual for patients with liver and gallbladder conditions*.

Cholesterol and coronary heart disease

Infections were once the most frequent cause of death. With an increasing standard of living and the connected change of nutrition and lifestyle, as well as the introduction of antibiotics, cardiovascular diseases have become the most common cause of death. In the early 20th century, Dr. med. Maximilian Bircher-Benner reported that widespread and increasingly poor nutrition and lifestyles caused an increase of all 'diseases of civilisation. diseases.[94] In 1910, Adolf Windaus, later a Nobel prize laureate, documented that arteriosclerotic plaques consisted mainly of cholesterol. In the mid 20th century, the hypothesis of the famous nutritionist Ancel Keys was given great attention. According to Keys, the exponential increase of cardiovascular diseases had been caused by the fatty nutrition composed of an abundance of meat, dairy products, eggs and butter. Keys claimed that the high cholesterol continent in nutrition caused arteriosclerosis, a claim that is disputed today. Keys' work led to the prescription of low-cholesterol diets and the production of a large range of cholesterol-reduced industrial products and margarines, and even the frequent prescription of cholesterol-reducing medication (statins).

Today about 25 million people worldwide regularly take cholesterol-reducing preparations. These medicines generate the highest turnover in the pharmaceutics industry, at USD 27 billion per year.[95] However, the frequency of cardiovascular diseases has barely moved since then. It was later shown that the low risk for cardiovascular diseases among the Japanese population adjusted to the high American risk once the Japanese had immigrated to the USA and adjusted to the local lifestyle and nutrition.

As a consequence, the entire range of risk factors was assembled: age, gender (male), smoking, diabetes mellitus, hypertension, obesity and a sedentary lifestyle. Studies carried out by the statin manufacturers documented that high-risk candidates for heart attack could reduce the heart attack risk slightly by taking a statin regularly. Only in the past few years has a certain life-extending effect of taking statins been demonstrated. However, this was only the case in part of the studies performed, and was limited to middle-aged, high-risk male patients. There are persons with a version of the LDL cholesterol receptor gene who naturally have lower LDL cholesterol values. Their heart attack risk is 23 % lower.[96]

Towards the end of the 20th century, more value was placed on the ratio of high-density lipoprotein HDL to low-density lipoprotein, since it had been proven that high LDL and low HDL led to a higher risk of heart attack.

It was not until the early 21st century that it was found that the cause of arteriosclerosis was not LDL cholesterol, but rather that LDL cholesterol is oxidised on its way to the tissues because of poor nutrition and oxidative stress. It was found that the foam cells of the arteriosclerosis foci contained only oxidised LDL cholesterol.

Unsaturated omega-3 and omega-6 fatty acids are strong antioxidants. They effectively protect the LDL cholesterol on its path into the tissues from oxidation, something that saturated fatty acids cannot do sufficiently.

In the USA, the National Cholesterol Education Program (NECP) regularly issues recommendations for the treatment of patients with high cholesterol. The Deutsche Gesellschaft für Kardiologie (DGK) uses them as a reference.

The NECP III distinguishes between the risk groups: 1) Patients who suffer from arteriosclerosis in their coronary vessels or from diabetes. Their heart attack risk for the next 10 years is estimated to be at least 20 %. 2) Patients with at least two risk factors (e.g.

hypertension and high LDL cholesterol).
3) Patients with fewer than two risk factors.[97]

The following risk factors today
Smoking
Hypertension above 140/90 mmHg,
HDL cholesterol below 1.03 mmol/ml (40 mg/100 ml),
family history of coronary heart disease, direct ancestors: men under the age of 55, women under the age of 65
Age: men over the age of 45, women over the age of 55.

The following general recommendations currently apply:

Risk group 1:
At LDL cholesterol above 2.58 mmol/l (100 mg/dl): change of lifestyle
At LDL cholesterol above 3.36 mmol/l (130 mg/dl): statin medication

Risk group 2:
At LDL cholesterol above 3.36 mmol/l (130 mg/dl): change of lifestyle
At LDL cholesterol above 4.12 mmol/l (160 mg/dl): statin medication

Risk group 3:
At LDL cholesterol above 4.12 mmol/l (160 mg/dl): change of lifestyle and statin medication
At LDL cholesterol above 4.91 mmol/l (190 mg/dl): statin medication

The following lifestyle changes are recommended:

Nicotine abstinence
Reduction of animal fats (saturated fatty acids below 7 % of the overall energy) and cholesterol in food
Weight reduction
Using oils with polyunsaturated fatty acids
More exercise

This procedure is certainly insufficient, since it has only led to a minimal reduction of cardiovascular diseases.

The problem of statin medication
Critics note that recommendations based on the cholesterol hypothesis often lead to healthy persons prophylactically subjecting themselves to risky medication. The connection between cholesterol level and risk of coronary heart disease is low only in humans.
Cholesterol is an important part of the cell membrane and one of the most common and necessary substances in the body. Cholesterol is very important for the brain metabolism. Therefore the body regulates this substance by producing it, not by taking it in with food. The consequences of forcing the body to reduce cholesterol synthesis (statins) or increase excretion (cholestyramin) are very difficult to foresee. Only in men up to 45 years of age does the LDL cholesterol level correlate with the number of coronary heart diseases, even in family-related hypercholesterolemia, where there are still very high LDL cholesterol values even at that age. It has never been proven that an increased LDL level causes heart attacks. A high LDL cholesterol value is not connected to a reduction of life expectancy, at least not in older persons.[98, 99] A meta-analysis published in 1998 covering all present autopsy studies (examinations on deceased persons) has shown that persons whose medical history reflects high LDL cholesterol levels do not have to undergo more arteriosclerotic changes than those with normal LDL cholesterol levels.[100]

The problem of reducing cholesterol by medication with statins
The medication group of statins reduces the cholesterol level in the blood by inhibiting synthesis of the enzyme HMG-Co-reductase in the body. The body needs this enzyme to produce cholesterol, the

synthesis of which continually adjusts to demand in the liver and intestinal mucosa. Statins prevent this adjustment. Since the cells need enough cholesterol for the cytoplasmic membranes and their metabolism, the membranes produce additional receptors for LDL cholesterol when taking statins, in an attempt to receive enough LDL cholesterol. Because of the numerous receptors, increased amounts of LDL cholesterol are absorbed from the blood, thereby reducing the LDL level. However, arteriosclerosis is not caused by LDL cholesterol, but by its oxidation. Oxidised cholesterol can neither be used to stabilise the cytoplasmic membranes, nor for hormone formation, nor for synthesis of bile acids. Oxidised cholesterol deposits in the arterial walls as slag, where it is recognised as a foreign body, so that the immune system will try in vain to remove it by scavenger cells (macrophages). The artificial reduction of the overall cholesterol and LDL cholesterol levels by statins does not remove the oxidised LDL cholesterol, but produces a noticeable lack of urgently needed cholesterol for all tissues in the body. This is documented by the less-than-convincing effect of such medicines in the prevention of cardiovascular diseases and their consequences, and the great potential for partially life-threatening side effects. Even though this is relatively rare, statins do have very severe side effects, sometimes even fatal.

Statins, pregnancy and lactation
If a woman takes statins during pregnancy, the medicine will most likely cause severe malformations in the development of the brain and formation of the limbs of her child, very similar to those of thalidomide.[101] At low cholesterol levels, below 4.1 mmol/l (160 mg/dl), small and premature babies are more common than at higher values.[102] Breast milk contains 25 mg cholesterol/100 ml and cow's milk only 12 mg/100 ml. It is suspected that this is the reason why breastfed children have a higher intelligence quotient in later life, since cholesterol is very important for brain development.

Statins and memory
Numerous studies have documented that LDL cholesterol levels are correlated with memory performance and other cognitive skills. An artificial reduction of the LDL cholesterol level by medication, reducing the amount of this substance taken from the liver to the brain, will significantly reduce memory performance and attention. The connections (synapses) between the nerve cells of the brain (neutrons) are continually converted and adjusted to the mental requirements. It has been documented that the cholesterol in the brain plays an essential role in the formation of these synapses. Formation of synapses is decisive for memory and the ability to learn. Statins reduce the cholesterol level not only in the blood, but also in the brain. Specialised medical literature contains numerous cases of total memory loss in direct connection with cholesterol-reducing medication.[103, 104]

Statins and the risk of stroke
The Framingham study (the largest cohort study) and a meta-analysis of 45 recent cohort studies (with a total of 450,000 patients under observation and more than 13,000 cases of stroke) showed no interrelation between cholesterol level and the risk of stroke for those aged over 45. In patients younger than 45, the cholesterol values were higher in those who had had a stroke than in other patients.[105] In other studies, women with a higher cholesterol level and aged younger than 45 had a slightly higher prevalence of stroke, while those older than 45 had a significantly lower prevalence of stroke than women with a lower cholesterol level.[106]

Hypertension is an important risk factor for stroke. It is suspected that the documented reduction of stroke risk by 17 %

from statin medication is not the result of a reduction in cholesterol, but because the medication reduces blood pressure.[107]

Reduction of cholesterol levels by statins and risk of cancer

Many studies examine the influence of a reduction of cholesterol levels by statins on the risk of cancer. Studies that document a much higher risk are opposed by those that show no influence or suggest a reduction of the cancer risk. The results are clearly very contradictory.

Reduction of cholesterol levels and depression

Among young women, depression was twice as common at overall cholesterol levels under 4.14 mmol/l (160 mg/dl) than in women with higher levels.[108] Among 236 older patients with depression, those who took statins had an 80 % higher risk of relapses.[109] In a placebo-controlled study among 70-year-old patients, the mood of those who were treated with cholesterol-reducing statins was significantly negatively impaired, as compared to those without statin therapy.[110] As the cholesterol levels are reduced by statins, the patients suffer nightmares more often.[111,112]

Statin medication and physical performance

It has been shown that it is much harder to improve the physical performance of the heart and muscles in patients who take statins than in those who do not. Reasons named are not only the muscle pain caused by the statins, but also inhibition of the formation of the enzyme citrate synthetase in the mitochondria (the power plants of the cells) by the statin, so that the aerobic glucose breakdown for energy production in the cells is inhibited.[113]

Reduction of cholesterol levels by statins and potentially fatal side effects

The most severe side effects of statins include toxic myopathies. This is a change of the structure and function of the skeletal muscles. The most severe form of toxic myopathy is rhabdomyolysis, which causes the fatal destruction of the striated muscle of the heart and all motor muscles. By 2003, 3,350 such fatalities due to statin medication had been reported. Only in 2012 were the manufacturers of statins required to include the risk of rhabdomyolysis (IMNM: immune-mediated necrotizing myopathy) in their package inserts.[114]

Critics of the widespread campaigns and the sometimes ill-considered treatment of many millions of healthy persons with statins note that the ratio of defective prophylactic and therapeutic effects to the potential of partially life-threatening side effects and risks, as well as costs (billions), is not in correspondence with sensible or logical medical action. In fact, the fatalities due to cardiovascular diseases in Germany have declined very little.

The importance of proteins and amyloidosis

Excessive consumption of animal protein, especially from meat and cheese, is another important partial cause of arteriosclerosis. Amyloidosis refers to the depositing (slagging) of abnormal (degenerative) proteins in the intracellular substance, the basic substance of the soft connective tissue. Such deposits can generally happen in any type of body tissue. Generalised forms of amyloidosis are rare deposits throughout the body that can be congenital or caused by chronic diseases. They occur in about 1 out of 100,000 persons per year.

The degenerative proteins are folded abnormally as molecules, forming fine fibrils that destroy the tissues, e.g. in the brain in the case of Alzheimer's disease. Amyloid contains certain amino acids that occur less in plant-based proteins but are particularly rich in meat, cheese and eggs.

Amyloidosis may occur in the large aortas of any person in later life. An autopsy study of the aortas of 84 persons showed amyloid deposits in the aorta in all but one patient aged over 50.[115] This was confirmed in a number of further examinations[116, 117, 118] and shows that high consumption of both animal fats and animal proteins contributes to arteriosclerosis.

A person weighing 70 kg requires no more than 50 to 60 g of protein/day with a balanced amino acid content. This supply is very important for cell replacement in the body. Excess additional protein can no longer be used for cell replacement. The body must first break down the protein molecules into its components, the amino acids; then it must remove the main group chemically, turning them into short-chained carbohydrates that it can turn into glucose molecules to use as energy substrate in the mitochondria.

Since this entire conversion process in the metabolism is very uneconomic, the calorific energy of high-protein food produces one third of pure waste heat that the body cannot use otherwise. This waste heat, which can be felt as a warming sensation after a protein-rich meal, was inaccurately called the 'specific dynamic effect' by Berlin physiologist Max Rubner in 1900. It is easy to mistake this senseless heat development for usable energy. When breaking down excess proteins, the metabolism partially produces toxic degradation products that cannot be excreted quickly enough and that will put stress on the kidneys. They will deposit in the basic substance of the soft connective tissue and some become amyloids. For this reason, the protein economy in food is very important for preventing arteriosclerosis and degenerative disorders.

The importance of carbohydrates and sugar for arteriosclerosis

Carbohydrates are nutrients that are made up mainly of molecules built from hydrocarbon chains.

A number of researchers confirm that carbohydrates too play a major role in the development of arteriosclerosis. Many test results support this finding in regard to industrial sugar, white-flour products and other refined carbohydrates in abundance today.

The starch of white superfine flour is split very quickly into sugar molecules. The saccharose of cooking sugar, fructose and lactose are also split into simple sugar molecules and immediately converted to glucose, which is then broken down completely into carbon dioxide and water to produce the cell energy in a number of breakdown steps (the chemical 'respiratory chain' in the mitochondria). This produces energy-rich phosphates, which are used as energy substrate in any number of chemical-conversion steps. Excess carbohydrates that are not needed for covering energy demand are converted into fat and stored in the fatty tissue.

We distinguish between simple carbohydrates (such as the different types of sugar) and complex carbohydrates, whose sugar content is polymerised and bound to many other molecules so that the sugar can only be removed after great effort by the digestive enzymes.

Industrial sugar, white-flour products and other refined carbohydrates can contribute decisively to metabolic imbalances that provoke storage of degenerated fat and proteins and LDL cholesterol in the basic substance of the tissues. Refined and concentrated sugar removes vitamins and impairs the task of the organism to properly utilise fat and protein. Sugar is utilised very differently when integrated into a natural composite of fruits, wholemeal and vegetables.

It is essential to dispense with the habitual enjoyment of refined sugar and white-flour food and return to whole cereals and naturally sweet sources (e.g. fruit, honey).

The ingestion of food will increase the glucose level in the blood until it drops again by the excretion of insulin and by the utilisation of the glucose in the cells. The speed, strength and duration at which food increases the blood-sugar level is called the glycaemic index (GI), which figuratively corresponds to the area under the rising curve of the blood glucose. The glucose content in the food to be tested is calculated to determine the GI. Then the rising curve for a specific amount of this food is measured and compared to that of the same test quantity of pure glucose.

A high glycaemic index means that eating this food will produce a quick, high blood-sugar increase that will cause excretion of a large amount of insulin for quick return of the blood sugar level to the standard value. After consuming a food with a low glycaemic index, the blood sugar will increase later, more slowly and for longer, which will require a much lower amount of insulin. Foods with a high glycaemic index, such as foods composed of white superfine flour and refined sugar, contain glucose in quickly available form and put us at risk of diabetes mellitus.

The glycaemic load (GL) of food is calculated by taking its glycaemic index (GI) and multiplying it by its content of pure carbohydrates. Foods with a high glycaemic index and high glycaemic load strongly impair the fat metabolism. They produce an increased triglyceride level and a lower HDL cholesterol level.[119, 120, 121] In a study involving 75,521 women over 10 years, those who ate foods with high glycaemic loads (GL) suffered heart attacks much more often.[122] Heart attacks were even more common in those women who were also obese and in whom insulin resistance had already been documented.[123]

Refined superfine flours contain more starch and less dietary fibre, fewer secondary plant substances and essential oil with polyunsaturated fatty acids. Several comparative studies have shown that an increased ingestion of wholemeal will effectively lower heart-attack risk.[124, 125, 126, 127, 128]

The importance of vegetarian nutrition in the prevention of coronary heart disease

Food containing folic acid is vegetable food with many green leaves. A deficit of folic acid is connected to an increased homocystein level, which is considered an indication of increased infarction risk. Many studies have been performed to document that a high content of folic acid in food considerably reduces the risk of heart attack and apoplexy.[129, 130, 131, 132, 133, 134, 135, 136] In some of these studies, vitamin B_6 was added to the folic acid. These two vitamins are mostly found in fresh, raw fruit and vegetable food.

The effect of almonds and nuts to counter arteriosclerosis

Several prospective studies have consistently shown that eating unroasted almonds and nuts protects from coronary heart disease. Nuts do not increase weight. They contain only mono- and polyunsaturated oils and lower the levels of LDL cholesterol in the blood in a harmless, natural manner.[137, 138, 139, 140, 141, 142, 143]

The effect of fruits and vegetables on arteriosclerosis

Plant foods do not contain cholesterol but they do have cholesterol-reducing ingredients (secondary plant substances). The saponins of the legumes reduce cholesterol naturally and harmlessly by reducing its resorption in the intestine. The primary bile acids are synthesised from cholesterol by the liver and emitted through the biliary ducts into the intestine for fat resorption, after which they return to the liver through the portal vein as fat mycelia (enterohepatic cycle). Only a small part of the primary bile acids is converted into secondary bile acids by the bacterial flora and excreted. The saponins increase this extrusion by saponification and thus effectively reduce cholesterol. Beans and Lucerne/alfalfa are particularly rich in saponins. The addition of 40 g of heat-treated Lucerne/alfalfa seeds three times a day with meals reduces the cholesterol level by 18 %. Cold-pressed plant oils contain phytosterins. They reduce cholesterol levels in various ways.[144] Tocotrienols in whole-grain seeds of rye, barley, oats, palm oil, oat oil and barley oil inhibit the synthesis of cholesterol effectively and in a harmless manner. The allicin in garlic moderately inhibits cholesterol synthesis in the liver. Allicin in garlic, carotenoids in fruits and vegetables, vitamins C and E and anthocyanins in aubergines reduce LDL cholesterol and prevent its oxidation.

The antioxidative effect of vegetarian raw food, the importance of secondary plant substances

Only vegetarian food, and particularly raw food, is rich in substances with a pharmacological effect, called secondary plant substances. We refer here to the Bircher-Benner manual no. 4: *Manual of fresh juices, raw vegetables and fruit dishes*.

Many epidemiological studies show connections between oxydative stress with a weakened antioxidative system and a high risk of cancer, cataract, cardiovascular disease, arteriolosclerosis, multiple sclerosis and other degenerative conditions.[144] A diet high in fruit and vegetables, particularly in the form of raw vegetables, is the most effective protection from degenerative conditions. The recommendations of the German Nutrition Society (Deutsche Gesellschaft für Ernährung, or DGE) have been adjusted in accordance with this insight. An essential share of this effect is due to the content in secondary plant substances, particularly in raw fruit and vegetables. Flavonoids are partially lost when fruits and vegetables are peeled, but not when they are cooked. However, the protective effect of carotenoids (xanthines) is entirely lost in cooking.[145] We refer here to the Bircher-Benner manuals no. 4: *Manual of fresh juices, raw vegetables and fruit dishes*; no. 24: *Manual for prevention of dementia and Alzheimer's disease*; and no. 1: *Manual for patients with multiple sclerosis*.

The acute crises in cardiovascular diseases are always connected to the thromboembolic events, since the blood of many patients is viscose and clots easily. Raw onions and garlic are especially effective in preventing blood clots, as are flavonoid-containing citrus fruits and fruits in general because of their high polyphenol content. These foods inhibit the aggregation of blood platelets (thrombocyte aggregation inhibition). In garlic containing ajoene, this effect is strongest and comparable to the effective strength of aspirin (acetyl salicylic acid).[146] Garlic extract and powder are not effective here. The sulphides ajoene in garlic and allicin in fresh onion and garlic inhibit thrombocyte aggregation (the sticking together of blood platelets) by inhibiting (catalysing) enzymes that form thromboxane, just like flavonoids in fruits and vegetables and sulphides in onion plants. Similar effects on blood-platelet aggregation have been documented for polyphenols in the outer layers of fruit and vegetables. In an epidemiological study, patients with cardiovascular disease who had the highest flavonoid intake through citrus and fruits showed the lowest mortality rate.[147]

Flavonoids are lost largely through the peeling of fruit and vegetables and also partially through storage. However, flavonoids withstand cooking. Even though the positive effects of fruit and vegetables are widely recognised today, it is surprising that epidemiological examinations of the importance of fruit and vegetables to reduce the risk of arteriosclerosis and infarction have been performed only recently.[148] Those published so far consistently confirm a high degree of protection of plant food, particularly when ingested as vegetarian fresh food (raw food).[149,150,151,152,153,154,155,156]

The importance of wholemeal cereals

Wholemeal instead of white or grey superfine meal protects to a large extent from coronary heart disease and brain infarctions (apoplexy).[157, 158, 159]

Bircher-Benner's healing diet and order therapy

All of these examinations confirm our more than 100 years' experience in the therapeutic treatment of cardiovascular diseases. Arteriosclerosis with its tragic consequential diseases can not only be prevented, but often even healed. Important Individual studies also confirm the reversibility of arteriosclerosis through diets which are very similar to ours. As we have seen, the causes of arteriosclerosis are complex. The focus is on: poor nutrition; excessive ingestion of animal products (e.g. meat, sausage, pickled sliced meat, barbecue kebabs, dairy products, eggs and cheese); denatured, industrially degraded ready-made products; alcohol, irritants (e.g. overly strong coffee, black tea, energy drinks); overly sweet cereal bars and 'snack foods', sugary drinks, sugary yoghurt, sugary jams; white bread, refined-flour foods, pastry, sugar pastry and chocolate; hamburgers, French fries, sweet ketchups, Minipicks, paprika chips; and much more.

We have seen that LDL cholesterol is vital for supplying all tissues with cholesterol to stabilise the cell membranes and their metabolism, and for hormone synthesis. We have seen how much people today suffer from oxidative stress because of poor nutrition, overwork, bullying and relationship problems, a disorderly lifestyle, lack of sleep, electro smog and medication. We have seen that the lack of antioxidants due to the widespread deficit of secondary contents from plant-based fresh food and due to the deficit of polyunsaturated vegetable oils puts too big a burden on the abilities of the antioxidative system and enzymes to counter oxidation, causing LDL cholesterol to oxidise and turn rancid. We have seen that only oxidised LDL cholesterol will deposit in the intima of the arteries and, because of its high amount, block the receptor path of cholesterol breakdown, since the macrophages are unable to remove it and turn into inactivated foam cells that indicate the beginnings of arteriosclerotic depositing and destruction of the arterial walls.

The reduction of the arteriosclerosis risk is also supported by a rich supply of alkaline minerals, specifically potassium and magnesium, in green and bulbous vegetables, wholemeal, nuts and potatoes. When sodium (table salt) and calcium are kept low, the effects are all the better. Magnesium increases phosphate turnover. Food rich in meat and protein inhibits magnesium intake, while vegetarian fresh food is rich in potassium and magnesium and provides all minerals at an ideal ratio and in keeping with bioavailability.

In industrial nations, human food intake calculated in calories is about half more than the body needs. Appetite is increased by obesity, lack of vital substances, appetising industrial additives, coffee, irritants from roasting, frequent snacks and frequent intake of sugar and fast carbohydrates.

The nutrition change suggested in this book regulates appetite within a few weeks, so that the pathological yearnings will cease. Reducing the food volume by one-third and doing without interim meals and snacks not only relieves and economises the metabolism, but also essentially contributes to normalising body weight, reducing blood pressure, healing arteriosclerosis and reducing the risk of cardiovascular disease.

The instructions and treatment plans in this book have been designed to help in achieving this target. Natural nutrition rich in fresh food and composed of unrefined and tastily prepared dishes helps reduce the widespread incentive to eat too often and too much and the demand for stimulating drinks and irritants.

Medical experience shows that the typical arteriosclerosis patient is a person who 'can eat anything', who especially likes fatty foods, and who likes to 'let himself go' at the table. Nothing keeps him from joining in the common eating, drinking, smoking and stimulating habits with plenty of rich, tart food, meat, confectionery and preserves. There are also those who eat simply but ingest snacks of all kinds between meals. Binge eating and obesity are usually present in such cases, and so is a considerable consumption of irritants, alcoholic drinks, sweets, frequent abuse of laxatives, painkillers and soporifics. The result is degenerated intestinal flora and slow, impaired digestion, often accompanied by a weak liver, irritability and inner unrest. Some patients seem unable to get away from compulsive excursions into town (instead of walks in the forest and fields), are easily depressed after anger and disappointment, and tend to view their environment with distrust or withdrawal. In such a situation, a good measure of patience, skill and confidence among family, doctors, nurses and therapists is necessary. Arteriosclerosis therapy requires intelligence, understanding and cooperation on the part of the patient.

If started in time, before the organs have been destroyed, arteriosclerosis can be healed by a vegan diet rich in fresh food, as described in this book, as long as the diet is adhered to. The patient must rigorously begin the diet stages of fresh juices and raw food, and continue the diet very diligently for many months. This will slowly reduce the arteriosclerotic narrowing in the arteries and improve the blood supply.[160, 161] The improved intestinal flora helps regulate appetite and body weight. Bacteria from the large intestine produce vitamin B_{12}. Nevertheless, the vitamin B_{12} supply must be monitored for a strict vegan raw food diet.[162, 163] Vitamin B_{12} can also be absorbed via sea buckhorn pulp or natural yeast extract. For those already suffering from angina pectoris, cooperation with a cardiologist is particularly important during the dietary treatment. It will help to remember that a strict healing diet is necessary until the arteriosclerosis foci have been removed, and that the very tasty nutrition which will keep the patient healthy can be used afterwards. It takes great intelligence and good will and it is worthwhile to persevere. After a few weeks, an immense relief will be noticed, even in cases of 'intermittent claudication' (claudication intermittens due to constricted leg arteries). The walking distance until the cramp-like pain occurs will increase over time. The blood pressure will often take a longer time to drop considerably, so that blood-pressure-lowering medication can only be reduced slowly and under medical supervision and review of the condition of the coronary vessels. Only then will the threat from the complications of arteriosclerosis, the disasters of stroke or heart attack, be over.

Hypertension

The development of arteriosclerotic changes in the circulatory system will always increase blood pressure and overall tension. This can be easily understood from what has been explained thus far. This increase in blood pressure, however, may remain within moderate limits that are still considered normal. The Inuit Indians of eastern Greenland provide a good example of this. These hunters develop arteriosclerosis very early and will show dangerously high degrees of arterial changes starting in the third decade of life. The nutrition of Inuits is scarce and usually uncooked, but very rich in animal protein and fat. Nevertheless, their blood pressure barely exceeds what Westerners consider normal (because it corresponds to the average in middle age and does not lead to any outward symptoms). When compared to other primitive peoples who do not live from hunting but from farming, the Inuits' blood pressure difference is considerable. We can see that there appears to be a different standard that is lower and does not increase with age. This is the standard we believe is the true one, while the higher standard used by the specialist world would be the Western standard. It has not been determined where the true blood pressure and cholesterol level standard actually lies.

To the contrary, a vegetarian religious order and a poor African population eating little protein and fat showed neither arteriosclerotic degeneration nor increase of cholesterol levels. However, they did show increased blood pressure on average, probably because of excessive consumption of table salt.

The ice dwellers of eastern Greenland lead a primitive lifestyle that poses extreme challenges to the adaptability of the human organism in the middle of an environment that is very hostile to life. Their nutrition is close to nature. However, it is mostly made up of the fatty meat of animals not kept on farms but living in the wild. If they were eating farm animals, these Inuit would surely have become extinct long ago.

Blood pressure rises as a life-saving necessity, an emergency measure by a damaged organism. Otherwise the organs would not receive an adequate supply of blood. In healthy persons, blood pressure is kept at a normal level. After any deviation, this regulating mechanism will return the blood pressure to a normal level. Special occasions in life that require intense performance increases of the body. These coincide with a temporary increase in blood pressure. High-performing organs must be supplied with more blood, though not for too long. Normal levels must always be returned to. If they are not, recovery is impossible and the heart and circulation 'wear out'. Particularly during sleep, the blood pressure drops to a minimum.

The regulation of blood pressure appears to be relatively effective in humans, just as that of the cholesterol level; otherwise the immense problem of hypertension diseases would not exist.

Of course, sustained blood pressure increase may also be a side effect of various organic diseases. A doctor will first have to determine this on a case-to-case basis. Only 5 % of all cases show such an organic cause, however. Ninety-five percent suffer from actual hypertension (essential hypertension). In these cases, the only reason for failure of regulation is excessive stress.

Psychosomatic partial causes are often present, due to persistent insults, anger, fearfulness, anxiety, fury, and any sustained excess mental stress. Other important cause are general excessive stress and exhaustion. Where people no longer experience any deepened relationship with others and with themselves in the hectic pace of everyday life or where, contrary to their actual nature, they subject themselves to the permanent stress of performing tasks that are without sense for themselves and others, where they are no longer up to meeting the diversity of their tasks, experience setbacks and disappointment, have to put up with counter-pressure and emotional tensions, all of this continually repeated, blood pressure may, even without other causes, increase temporarily at first and constantly later.

A condition of permanent stress in this sense leads to permanent over-excitation of the sympathetic nervous system and increased adrenaline levels. More and more business executives and managers are living at this stage of the burnout syndrome. Ensnared in the principle of profit maximisation, they often spend years or decades living with permanent tension and without experiencing the deeper sense and satisfaction of their actual skills and talents. There is a good reason why hypertension is called the 'Managers' disease'.

Furthermore, the inherited constitution plays a role as well, as blood pressure increases are early and strong for some people and late and weak for others.

It can also happen that the regulation can be so exhausted that blood pressure paradoxically drops. A patient with a blood pressure disorder must learn how to live with his heart, rather than against his deeper sense of life.

However, it is important not to lose sight of what is essential. When food is so constituted as to prevent arteriosclerosis and hypertension, temporary excitement and mental stress often have little or no effect in the creation of hypertension.

When there is constant overload of the kidneys from food too rich in protein, the organism will increase blood pressure to enforce excretion of the relevant breakdown products.

Food rich in meat will increase this effect, from the irritating effect of the extractive substances, such as they are extracted for meat broth, and often too from roasting by-products. Added to this is the additional stress on the liver from the excess protein in the food. Other causes of hypertension are suppurate foci in the dental roots, the tonsils or endotoxins of putrefactive agents of an impaired intestinal flora due to the protein overload. Thus blood pressure may increase even in young persons. In smokers, the continuous stress on the body from carbon monoxide, nicotine, heavy metals and other toxins of cigarette smoke is very important. In order to calm the irritation produced by nicotine abuse, a smoker will chain smoke.

Experience shows that where meat dishes are prominent, spices and salt are also prominent. These will substantially damage the intestinal flora, causing obstipation and weight increase. Eating large quantities of salt alone will force the body to increase blood pressure.

Chronic hypertension will compress the fine blood vessels like a slow, perfidious vice, making them narrower and narrower, cramping and finally barely letting the blood flow pass. However, blood circulates in a closed system without a pressure valve, and blood pressure must increase unfailingly to ensure an adequate supply to the organs. If it rises too high and the vascular walls lose their suppleness, they must be reinforced by additional connective tissue with collagen fibres. This is not possible without stiffening, so that the effect of the increasing pressure may cause bursting somewhere (e.g. in the brain, the heart, the kidneys or the eyes).

This development of hardening of the heart muscle, the arteries and arterioles (sclerotisation) may progress over years or decades and often shows no symptoms for a very long time. There are some persons who do not even suffer a headache at the very high blood pressure of 300 mm Hg. There are also those who feel very ill at a moderately increased blood pressure of 180 mm Hg. In any case, the continuous overload will sooner or later destroy the heart. The heart muscle reinforces itself with additional muscle layers (hypertrophy). The left atrium, however, will soon expand, so that the pacemaker centre, the sinus node and the excitation conducting system in the atrium muscle will fail. Thus excitation will start to circle quickly and senselessly in the atrium, causing it to vibrate instead of emptying into the ventricle. Atrial fibrillation often is the first complication of sustained hypertension which will destroy the body little by little with repeated embolisms.

Hypertension (above 130/90) is one of the main risk factors for arrhythmia, heart attack and stroke (apoplexy). The inside of the cells is rich in potassium, while the space between the cells is rich in sodium. Chemical sodium/potassium pumps maintain this difference (gradient) and thus determine the electrical potential of the cell membrane. The proportion of sodium to potassium is decisive for the regulation of blood pressure. This sodium/potassium gradient regulates liquid volume in the cells and the inter-cellular tissue, and permits transport of sugars and amino acids through the cell membrane into the cells. Transport of potassium ions into the cell and of sodium ions from the cell and the corresponding liquid transport thus determins blood volume and thus the blood pressure in the vessels. Blood pressure studies in different peoples with traditional lifestyles – the Khoi San in southern Africa, the Inuit in the Arctic, the Polynesians and the Central American native peoples – showed that average blood pressure values increase massively with the introduction of 'modern' nutrition with high sugar and salt content, preserved meat and fish, and other industrially processed foods.[164] Fibre-rich (fruit and vegetable) nutrition lowers blood pressure by means of various mechanisms.[165] Some dietary fibre is broken down by intestinal bacteria into short-chained fatty acids that lower blood pressure. Pectins are water-soluble dietary fibres in apples, bananas and citrus fruits with blood-pressure-reducing effects. Caffeine and theophylline from coffee and black tea displace adenosine from its receptors on the cells and thus increase blood pressure. At the brain neurons, adenosine will block the entrance of information into the brain cells (neurons) at overload of the nervous system to protect them from exhaustion. Caffeine blocks the adenosine receptors. Drinking coffee continually sabotages this important protective mechanism of the brain cells and thus causes them to become dangerously exhausted. Blood pressure reducing substances are isolated from garlic and leek preparations, including adenosine and allicin. This effect of fresh garlic can help to treat hypertension.

The blood pressure must vary within a certain bandwidth. Too high and too low blood pressure may both be harmful to vessels and organs. On the other hand, the blood pressure must be adjusted to demand during physical effort, e.g. an endurance run, but also in rest and sleep.

Blood pressure regulation

In the aorta, the carotid arteries and other large arteries in the neck and chest, there are pressure-sensitive cells called baroreceptors that continually measure the expansion of the arterial wall and thus the blood pressure, and report this to the blood pressure centre in the extended medulla of the brain stem (medulla oblongata) via vegetative nerve fibres of the sympathetic nervous system. If blood pressure increases too far, these impulses will inhibit the blood pressure centre. If the blood pressure is too low, the baroreceptor cells will reduce their impulses to the blood pressure centre, causing it to increase the frequency and ejection power of the heart via the sympathetic nerve fibres of the heart. The sympathetic nervous system also narrows the small arteries (arterioles) in the skin, the kidneys and the gastrointestinal tract. Both atria of the heart also have expansion receptors that affect the blood pressure centre. This kind of blood pressure regulation is used for momentary adjustment to stress and relaxation. Its effect is immediate.

Medium-term blood pressure regulation takes place via the kidneys. When the arterial pressure in one or both renal arteries drops, the kidneys will release the hormone renin into the blood stream. Renin activates the hormone angiotensin, which circulates in the blood and in turn constricts the arterioles throughout the body (vasoconstriction). This increase of vascular resistance increases blood pressure considerably. Healthy kidneys properly regulate the renin release. If the renal artery is narrowed by arteriosclerosis, the affected kidney will release renin continuously and sharply increase blood pressure on a permanent basis, since it is trying to retain its own blood supply.

Long-term blood pressure regulation takes place via the blood volume. If the arterial average pressure increases in the long term, the kidneys will reduce the blood volume by resorbing less sodium and water. The brain stem will also send signals to the posterior pituitary (neurohypophysis), signals that will cause it to release less anti-diuretic hormone than in normal conditions. The reduction of the antidiuretic hormone (ADH) in turn reduces the resorption of water in the collecting tubes of the kidneys, reducing blood volume and thus blood pressure quickly. Since the kidneys reduce renin release in order to decrease blood pressure, the angiotensin level will also fall.

Under the influence of angiotensin, the kidneys will produce the hormone aldosterone. This stimulates the cells of the renal tubules, increases the return of sodium with water from the urine into the blood, and in exchange releases more potassium into the urine. Less aldosterone lowers blood pressure. The expansion receptors of the atria also act on the kidneys through transmitter substances, to reduce blood pressure if an atrium is over-extended.

The blood pressure regulation therefore is very complex. It is not surprising that various influences and diseases will impair regulation, especially by a permanent increase of blood pressure, which will not return to normal levels during rest and sleep.

Hypertension arises from the same dietetic factors as arteriosclerosis, especially in the case of obesity. Thus the average blood pressure values of men and women increase with weight.[166, 167] The fatty tissue produces the hormone leptin, which acts on the appetite centre in the brain stem. If there is enough fatty tissue, the leptin level is higher and reduces appetite. Similar to the way insulin resistance is engaged by slagging off the basic substance of the soft connective tissue, thereby preventing insulin from reaching the cell membranes, the same phenomenon prevents the effect of leptin at the brain stem in obesity, so that the appetite will no longer be reduced and too much fatty tissue is stored.

The composition of bacteria of the intestinal flora depends on nutrition. It also influences body weight. The intestinal flora of obese persons contains mostly bacteria of the Firmicutes type, while weight reduction will increase the share of bacteroides. Bacteria-free non-obese mice into which the intestinal content of overweight mice was implanted would increase in weight in spite of reduced food intake.[168, 169, 170]

The fatty tissue of the abdomen and the entrails has a different metabolism from that of the limbs. If we do not move about, i.e. if we do not walk for at least an hour per day, abdominal fat will collect in the abdominal walls and the viscera. During the dietetic treatment of obesity, the body can only remove abdominal fat if we walk for one hour (or better, two) per day. The more abdominal fat is present, the more likely hypertension is to occur.

Too much table salt is a long-accepted partial cause of hypertension. Large quantities of table salt will stimulate the aldosterone release from the kidneys. Too much aldosterone will cause scarring of the muscle layers of the coronary arteries and the heart muscle, which will impair heart performance (myocardial fibrosis).[171] Low-salt food will reduce blood pressure clearly.[172, 173]

Today approx. 50 million people in the USA suffer from hypertension. Worldwide the number is estimated to be about 1 billion people, with much lower prevalence among vegetarians.[174] A meta-analysis of 258 scientific studies during the period 1900 – 2014 chosen according to strict criteria confirms that vegetarians have much lower blood pressure than omnivores.[175] In 1995, a randomised diet-controlled multi-centric study was published with 456 healthy persons with systolic blood pressure under 160 and diastolic blood pressure under 85 mm Hg (DASH-Study). The average blood pressure values in three comparable groups with three different diets were observed. The dietary group with rich vegetarian food had the lowest blood pressure values.[176]

In 2006, the American Heart Association published new recommendations for blood pressure treatment. It noted that the increased risk of cardiovascular diseases starts with blood pressure values that exceed 115/75. Today, for blood pressure of up to 159/99 mm Hg, medication is no longer recommended. Instead, recommendations go towards dietary therapy favouring plant-based food, a low salt diet and daily exercise. It is recommended that patients under medication follow these guidelines, even at higher values.[177] A subsequent examination of the DASH-diet showed that the contents of secondary plant substances (phytochemicals) in the diet-effective group were much higher than in others, especially flavonoids, beta-carotene, Betacryptoxanthine, lycopens, lutein, zeaxanthin and phytosterols. The important effect of these secondary plant substances for blood pressure regulation is only now beginning to be understood,[178] whereas the important effect of vegetarian diets had already been established in the USA in the 1970s[179] and rediscovered in recent years.[180, 181, 182, 183, 184] A major epidemiological study (INTERMAP Study) compared the effect of raw and cooked plant-based foods on blood pressure. Vegetables all had a blood pressure reducing effect, which was greatest in raw food. Raw tomatoes, carrots and spring onions have a very positive effect on the blood pressure. Cooked tomatoes, peas, celery and spring onions[185] have a similar effect. Walnuts, almonds and other nuts reduce blood pressure by means of their high content of polyunsaturated fatty acids. They do not increase weight. It has now been documented many times over that long-term vegan diets can heal hypertension.[186, 187, 188]

Pulmonary hypertension

There is another type of hypertension, this one related to pulmonary circulation, which in rare cases can be congenital (primary pulmonary hypertension). Usually this form of hypertension is acquired (secondary pulmonary hypertension) caused by a disease that increases the resistance of the arteries and thus the blood pressure in the pulmonary circulation. Usually the pulmonary artery has a blood pressure of 12–16 mm Hg. Pulmonary hypertension begins 25 mm Hg at rest and beyond 30 mm Hg under stress. From 30 to 40 mm Hg, the first clinical symptoms appear under stress in the form of exhaustion and shortness of breath. From 50 to 70 mm Hg, the output performance of the right heart reduces, since it is overexerted and weakened. The patients suffer from loss of consciousness (syncopes), angina pectoris, water retention in the legs, reduced circulation of the hands when cold (Raynaud's phenomenon) and persistent exhaustion. Arterial pressure in the pulmonary artery can exceed 100 mm Hg.

With pulmonary arterial hypertension, the pulmonary arteries narrow. Their muscles take on more mass and the connective tissue fibre layers of their walls thicken (sclerotisation). Consequently, the space inside the vessel narrows and the vessels scar and slowly stiffen. In this case, we speak of fixated lung hypertension, an irreversible condition. Such pulmonary arteries can also easily develop arteriosclerosis. The scarring of the pulmonary vessels also causes the lung tissue to scar, making it impossible to take in enough oxygen. The small bronchial tubes narrow so air is caught in the alveoli (lung emphysema). The patient suffers tormenting shortness of breath, first under effort and later also at rest. Idiopathic pulmonary hypertension is very rare (1–2 cases among one million persons). Various congenital heart problems lead to increased pressure in the pulmonary arteries. Luckily today, most of these can be removed by early surgical intervention. Almost all patients with a leaking mitral valve (mitral insufficiency) and about 60% of patients with a leaking aortal valve develop pulmonary hypertension because of backpressure in the pulmonary circulation (backward failure).

The most common cause of pulmonary hypertension, however, is chronic narrowing of the bronchial tubes, with increased scarring of the lung tissue (lung emphysema). The modern designation is COPD (chronic obstructive pulmonary disease. Once in a consultation, a 12-year-old girl told her mother, who had just smoked: 'Mama, smoking will suffocate you!' The mother was appalled, but the child was right and the mother was wrong. Either way, smokers are suffocated by lung cancer or other chronic obstructive lung diseases (lung emphysema). Contaminated air, the fine dust particles and nitrous oxides of diesel engines and heating, systems and chronic allergic bronchitides can cause chronically obstructive pulmonary diseases with pulmonary hypertension if not removed early. Rare causes include lung fibroses, AIDS, sarcoidose, sickle-cell anaemia and sclerodermia.

Treatment of hypertension with medication

This is a purely symptomatic treatment that must be continued, until the hypertension has been healed by dietary measures, to contain the risk of heart attack, stroke or bleeding from a burst artery (aneurysm haemorrhage, subarachnoid haemorrhage) until the cause has been healed.

If the cause is not treated by dietetic therapy, as is often the case, hypertension therapy with medication (like all therapies that suppress symptoms) will require increasing doses of the medicine. This can lead to a number of dangerous side effects.

Thanks to current scientific knowledge, we know that the following types of medication can influence blood pressure regulation:

ACE inhibitors
Substances that act where renin stimulates angiotensin were first found in snake venom. Numerous studies have led to the development of a substance group with names ending in -pril (Captopril, Enalapril, Lisinopril, Ramiplil and many others). These medicines are converted into the active substance in the body. ACE inhibitors reduce the cramped narrowing of the small arteries throughout the body and thus reduce blood pressure. An ACE inhibitor is usually the remedy of first choice. If the patient also suffers from diabetes the ACE inhibitor will to a degree protect the kidney by inhibiting protein release. For diets containing large quantities of table salt, ACE inhibitors show little effect. The most common side effect is an annoying, dry cough due to enrichment of bradykinin. ACE inhibitors increase the potassium level in the blood only slightly.

The skin may experience allergic reactions. Other side effects may be dangerous, but they are rare. Pregnant women should avoid ACE inhibitors, because these medicines can cause bone malformation in the foetus.

AT1 antagonists (sartans)
They inhibit the conversion of angiotensin I into the effective angiotensin II, thus acting in a similar manner as the ACE inhibitors. Their primary and side effects are similar, but there is less dry coughing. The results of large studies on the suspected increased risk of cancer have shown contradictory results.

Diuretics
If ACE inhibition is not enough, a drug is often added to inhibit the kidney's efforts to retain water. Drainage of the circulation leads to an undesired thickening of the blood (danger of thrombosis and embolisms) and reduces the ratio of sodium outside of the cells to the potassium within the cells (sodium/potassium gradient). This weakens the cell energy and often leads to fatigue and exhaustion. These medicines also have an undesired effect in the bile ducts of the liver, with corresponding side effects.

There are three groups of diuretics that target various parts of the renal tubules. Once a diuretic has been used, sodium and potassium levels must be monitored regularly by the general practitioner. Both are important, but potassium is especially critical. The side effects of diuretics are often underestimated and assigned to other causes.

Herbal diuretics
Vegan raw food naturally has a strong diuretic effect without side effects. It also improves viscosity of the blood by making the red blood corpuscles elastic again, enabling them to roll themselves up when flowing through the capillaries.
Goldenrod (Solidago virgaurea) and giant

goldenrod (Solidago gigantea) are extraordinary healing herbs. Apart from raw food, there is no other 'medicine' that is able to increase excretion of primary urine in the renal capillary loops. Other healing herbs include the large and small stinging nettle (urtica dioica and urea), weeping birch leaves (betula pendulans or alba), dandelion (taraxacum), orthosiphon leaves (orthosiphon stamineus or aristatus), field horsetail (equisetum arvensae) and spiny restharrow (ononis spinosa).

Before using any chemical diuretics, it is a good idea to try these much gentler but very valuable effects, in the form of a kidney-bladder tea mix or as spagyric essences.

Calcium antagonists
The calcium concentration inside the muscle cells of the heart and arterial walls usually is only one ten-thousandth of calcium concentration outside the cells. Outer stimuli open up chemical ducts, enabling calcium to enter the muscle cells and causing them to contract. This happens in hypertension, when the arterial vessels and the heart muscle are continually tense. Calcium antagonists inhibit this calcium inflow, reducing the heart rhythm and relaxing the heart muscles, the coronary vessels and the small pressure-regulating arteries throughout the body. The blood spreads into the capillary network, reducing vessel resistance, while the heart output drops, pushing the blood into the arteries with less force. The relaxation of the coronary arteries will cause more blood to enter the heart muscle.

There are three groups of medication types with this effect: Nifedipin-type, Verapamil-type and Diltiazem-type. Medicines of the Verapamil-type have a stabilising effect on the stimulus conduction system of the heart. Therefore, they are used to treat arrhythmia. The calcium antagonists are suitable when relaxation of the coronary vessels is important, e.g. in angina pectoris and hypertension in the pulmonary circulation. Side effects include oedema of the legs, bradycardia (or rarely tachycardia), reddening of the face, vertigo, headache, impotence, obstipation, swollen gums or allergic reactions. Calcium antagonists are often combined with ACE inhibitors, which reduces stroke risk and protects the kidneys from damage in case of diabetes. However, they offer less protection from heart attacks and heart failure than other substances.

Beta blockers
Hypertension or fear causes the sympathetic nervous system to produce an increased amount of the stress hormone adrenalin in the adrenal medulla, and noradrenaline at the synapses of the nervous system. With the heart, adrenaline increases the output force and heart frequency via beta-1 receptors, increasing blood pressure. Beta-2 receptors for adrenaline are present in the bronchial tubes, the uterus and the blood vessels, where this effect is not desired. Selective beta-1 receptor blockers have therefore been developed (Agenolol, Bisoprolol, Metoprolol, Nebivolol, Esmolol, Betaxolol). There also are beta-1 receptors in the kidneys, which release renin because of the effect of adrenaline. It is suspected that the blocking effect on the renin-angiotensin system is at the focus of the long-term effect of the beta blockers. They are used particularly during angina pectoris and after a heart attack and with chronic heart failure (cardiac insufficiency).

Beta blockers reduce the pulse at atrial fibrillation and stabilise the heart rhythm (they are also called II antiarrhythmics). They are now also used for many other conditions (e.g. hyperthyroidism, trembling, increased pressure inside the eye [glaucoma], migraines, anxiety, overpressure in the portal vein circulation due to cirrhosis of the liver) to prevent bleeding in the oesophagus, etc. They must not be combined with calcium antagonists or used in the case of asthma or chronically obstructive pulmonary disease, with bradycardia and in the case of certain disorders of excitation spreading in the heart. Slow pulse may cause dangerous falls due to syncopes (brief loss of consciousness), resulting in severe head injury.

Side effects of beta blockers are bradycardia, asthma, heart failure, fatigue, melancholy and impotence. Psoriasis and circulation impairment (in the case of constricted leg arteries) may grow worse.

Naturopathic blood-pressure-reducing medication

Squawroot (Rauwolfia serpentina)
This healing herb was already known three thousand years ago in India. It contains various alkaloids (including commonly known reserpine) with very strong effects and is therefore a prescription medicine. It lowers blood pressure by inhibiting the blood pressure centre in the brain stem (Medulla oblongata). At the same time, like Valium, it has a calming effect and alleviates fear. Thirty years ago, university medicine utilised a number of combinations of the rauwolfia alkaloid reserpine and chemical diuretics, which have gone out of fashion in spite of having proved their worth. Extracts of the entire plant have a better effect on blood pressure than the insulated reserpine. Rauwolfia must be dosed very carefully, since excessive doses may cause side effects similar to Parkinson's disease. Rauwolfia has been unjustly pushed into the background in the treatment of hypertension. In many cases, it has a better effect with fewer side effects than the chemical substances currently used. However, the dosage must be determined professionally and with care by the doctor.

Mistletoe (viscum album)
Mistletoe has proven very helpful for the treatment of light-to-moderate hypertension, and has barely any side effects. A tea according to the following recipe has proven particularly helpful:

> Rp. Herba visci albi
> Fol. et Flor. crataegi
> Fol melissae aa 100.0

Pour boiling water in a cup over 2 teaspoons of this mix in the morning and evening, let it steep for 10 minutes, and drink slowly. Crataegus (hawthorn) improves circulation in the coronary vessels, and balm calms the heart.

Folia Oleae (olive tree leaves)
Taken as a decoction or tincture, olive tree leaves lower blood pressure. However, this treatment may irritate the stomach and must therefore be taken after meals.

Angina pectoris

The name means 'narrow chest'. It is not a disease but a symptom, which is described as a pain in the region of the heart that comes in fits and is caused in part by a lack of circulation of the heart muscle. Usually the cause is an arteriosclerotic construction of one or several coronary vessels. This sharp pain is often felt in the middle of the anterior chest wall, and often even slightly to the right. When weaker it can radiate into both shoulders or the stomach area, and less often into the throat, lower jaw (Buddenbrook syndrome), and left arm down to the little finger or into the back. A dental root abscess may trigger or hide angina pectoris.

The pain is often accompanied by fear and sweating.

Stable angina pectoris

If these complaints always occur with the same kind of stress and in the same manner, the condition is called stable angina pectoris. This form is typical for arteriosclerosis of the coronary vessels (coronary sclerosis). In some patients, the pain will subside after a few minutes without rest. This phenomenon occurs because of by-pass circulation in the heart and must be treated just as urgently. Such attacks may be momentarily improved by nitro-glycerine, which expands the vessels. Prinzmetal's angina occurs without physical stress, rather as a stress symptom of general excessive tension, often in the scope of the 'managers' disease'. Angina pectoris attacks will subside just as quickly with a homoeopathic high-potency treatment of nitro-glycerine (glonoinum in the thousandth potency), just as effective as more substantial medication, with the benefit of acting more quickly and not causing any side effects (headache, flush). We give patients both as emergency medicines. If glonoinum does not work at once, nitro-glycerine should be used immediately. If this does not work quickly either, a heart attack may have occurred and the patient must be taken to an emergency room at once.

Unstable angina pectoris

The first occurrence of persistence of the pain is connected to a high risk of heart attack. Angina pectoris is also unstable if the pain increases slowly or if several fits grow worse or more frequent, or if they recur within two weeks of a heart attack. Unstable angina pectoris is caused by arteriosclerotic changes to the coronary vessels that have made a tear in the vascular wall. A blood clot (thrombus) may form from this and can occlude the vessel, thereby causing a heart attack. One form of unstable angina pectoris occurs when the victim is lying down at night, since the venous return flow will overload a weakened heart when lying down.

The CSS classification of cardiology distinguishes four severities: 1) Occurring only during fast, severe stress. 2) Occurring when walking quickly or climbing stairs or after meals; at taking more than one stair at a time or from a walking distance of 100 m onwards, at cold temperatures or under emotional stress. 3) Clear limitation of physical activity, when walking less than 100 metres or climbing stairs up one floor at normal speed. 4) Angina pectoris at rest and at low stress.

Germany sees about 300,000 hospital admissions every year for angina pectoris, the most common reason for emergency admission. During the attack, absolute rest should be observed, with the upper body raised at an angle of 30° and nitro-glycerine administered to the patient.
If the fit does not end within 15 minutes, an emergency doctor must be brought in and an ECG (electrocardiogram) administered. Nitro-glycerine releases nitro-oxygen (nitrous oxide, NO), which expands vessels significantly. Nitro-glycerine has no effect on pain from a heart attack. In this case, treatment of the infarction will be started at once.

Prevention and treatment of heart attack

With regard to both stable and unstable angina pectoris, timely treatment of the causes as specified in this book is decisive for the prevention of heart attack. A cardiac catheter examination often permits insertion of a stent into one or several constricted vessels. The stent is a last-minute emergency solution, rather than actual healing, since the locations that have been treated with a stent are much more likely to close up again.

Heart attack

Heart attack is one of the most common causes of death in industrial countries. In England and Hungary, there are 500 infarctions per 100,000 residents per year. In Scandinavia there are 400, in Germany 300 and in France 200–300. In Switzerland, the Mediterranean region and Japan there are fewer than 100 infarctions per 100,000 residents per year. The frequency of infarctions in Germany fell during the period 2000–2011, from 67,000 to 52,000.

Usually the infarction is caused by a blood clot in an arteriosclerotic bottleneck of a coronary vessel. The leading symptom is a sudden pain in the chest that may radiate into the shoulders, arms, lower jaw, back and upper abdomen, mostly on the left side, often coming with great fear and unrest, cold sweat and sometimes vomiting. One fourth of patients, however, feel little or nothing (silent infarction). Often at first there is dangerous arrhythmia or ventricular fibrillation. Any help will be too late.

If the typical pain persists for 20 minutes, this is called acute coronary syndrome. If the electrocardiogram (ECG) shows the typical ST-segment elevations, the diagnosis is clear (STEMI = ST-elevation myocardial infarction). However, there are also heart attacks without these elevations of the ST-segment in the ECG (NSTEMI = non ST-elevation myocardial infarction), which only a lab examination can distinguish from an unstable angina pectoris (Troponin CK_{MB} and others). If the destroyed hard muscle tissue reaches throughout the heart wall, the ECG will show a Q-wave after 12–24 hours. Death of the muscle will start after 15–30 minutes and happens from the inside outwards. Seventy-five percent of infarctions occur in places with only slight arteriosclerotic changes, and 25 % are due to tears of the plaque with blood clots (thrombus).

If the patient has suffered angina pectoris without arteriosclerosis (Prinzmetal's angina) for years, the cramping may also trigger an infarction. In rare cases, an inflammation of the heart (carditis) or tumour of the heart may cause an infarction.

If the right coronary artery (RCA) is affected, there will be a posterior myocardial infarction; if in the left coronary artery (LCA), an anterior myocardial infarction. Small infarctions occur when the vascular occlusion is in a distant, smaller vascular branch (large ones when a main trunk is affected). The left coronary artery is more branched out. Its main trunk (LCA) is short and immediately divides into a branch going around the heart (Ramus circumflexus, or RCX) and a branch going down the ventricles (ventricles) (Ramus interventricularis, or RIVA). An infarction in the circumflexus (RCX-branch) will cause a posterior myocardial infarction. An occlusion at the beginning of the RIVA-branch will cause a large anterior myocardial infarction. A far-distant occlusion of the RIVA branch will cause infarction in the separating wall between the two ventricles of the heart (septal infarction). Heart attacks are more common in the left coronary artery than in the right one.

The risk factors for heart attack

The greatest risk factors for infarction are considered to be: smoking, diabetes, obesity, hypertension, poor nutrition, a sedentary lifestyle and genetic predisposition. Factors such as constant anger, fury, insults, chronic stress and depression can also increase heart attack risk.

Many persons living in low-lying lands and cities suffer from vitamin D deficiency, especially since most no longer dare expose themselves to the sun without sunscreen. In winter, the UVB radiation from the sun that activates vitamin D cannot pass through the layers of fog. Vitamin D deficiencies will also increase the risk of heart attack. Therefore it is very important often to enjoy 20 minutes of exposure to the sun on both sides of the body without sunscreen in summer, with the head covered, and only then to go into the shade or use a fast-acting crystalline sunscreen cream. Persons of blood type A suffer infarctions more often, as do persons suffering from migraines with an aura. Myocardial infarctions are more common in socially disadvantaged areas and where there are high levels of fine dust pollution.

Caring for a heart attack victim

If a typical chest pain in the region of the heart continues in spite of nitro-glycerine, the ambulance must be called at once (call 112). The victim should never drive to the hospital himself. During the first hour, the danger of heart failure due to ventricular fibrillation is high. In places where there are many people, e.g. in the many 'shopping temples' and malls of our times, there are automated defibrillators that can be operated by laypeople. Using them may save lives.

While monitoring of the oxygen saturation of the blood, the ECG and blood pressure, specialists will administer nitro-glycerine, morphine, acetyl salicylic acid, heparin (to inhibit further blood clots) and clopidogrel. Then there will be an attempt to open up the clogged vessel. Therefore an ST-elevation myocardial infarction (STEMI) will have been treated in the ambulance by medication (streptokinase), in order to dissolve the thrombus (thrombolysis therapy). Once at the emergency room, an attempt to open up the occluded point again by inserting a cardiac catheter will be made (balloon catheter dilatation with stent insertion). Neither of these is possible in an NSTEMI myocardial infarction.

Once the first two hours have passed, the danger of ventricular fibrillation subsides. Today almost 90 % of patients survive a heart attack, including 75 % of those older than 75. Efficient organisation of emergency therapy for heart attack has cut mortality rates in half since 1980.[189]

Complications of heart attack

Permanent arrhythmia often follows as a consequence. If more than 30 % of the heart muscle is destroyed, circulatory failure is possible (cardiac shock). This is the second highest risk of death from myocardial infarction. Large infarction areas will bulge outwards into the pericardium and may burst there (cardiac tamponade) or blood clots may form in this kind of bulge, with a high risk of embolism (thromboembolism) if the clot reaches the brain or lung. If the septum is affected, a hole between the ventricles may form, which will lead to a dangerous acute overload of the right heart. A posterior myocardial infarction will cause part of the muscle (papillary muscle, which holds the flaps of the mitral valve) to die. The mitral valve must close the left ventricle against the atrium. If the mitral valve starts to leak, blood will flow back into the left atrium at each heartbeat. This puts too much stress on the atrium and ventricle, overstretching the wall of the left atrium and damaging the stimulus conducting system. This leads to arrhythmia. In the first two months after a heart attack, there is danger of developing pericarditis.

Prevention of heart attack

Many people rely on good emergency care and the technical possibilities of cardiologic meticulousness today. They live like everyone, without recognising the great tragedy and suffering that follow a heart attack. Suddenly one is old, sickly and weak, dependent on the diligent care of others, the general practitioner and the cardiologist. You will not know how long this is going to continue and how long you will still be able to live an acceptable life. Modern medical research has recently masterfully identified and explained the causes of coronary heart disease and arteriosclerosis in general. The prevention of such disasters is certainly possible. This book provides the knowledge and practical instruction to put your lifestyle and diet in order. The early reordering of lifestyle and diet is the only sustainably effective treatment for this disease. It takes courage and intelligence to foresee the tragedy of this disaster and to tackle the prevention of further problems.

Cardiac insufficiency or chronic heart failure

Hypertension usually becomes a lifelong disease, since the cause is never eliminated and the only treatment is through suppressive medication. The heart will adjust by thickening its muscles (hypertrophy). Thus it may be able to compensate for the overload for a shorter or longer period until it finally abandons the attempt. Then the heart muscle grows weak and the left atrium too is unable to fill the left ventricle properly, making it go slack. This will impair the conduction pathways, sooner or later causing atrial fibrillation. The failure of the output performance of the left heart (forward failure) causes fatigue and exhaustion, initially in the course of greater effort and later even with lighter efforts, until the heart is beating weakly and more quickly even at rest. This reduces oxygen supply throughout the body, a condition that is evident from a blue discolouration (cyanosis), particularly in the fingers, toes and lips. From the failing, weak left heart, the blood presses back into the lungs (backward failure), until water enters the lung tissue (lung oedema). This is made evident by a shortness of breath and rattling sounds when breathing, as well as liquid-foamy sputum, and requires immediate medical aid.

Pulmonary hypertension causes the muscle walls of the right ventricle to thicken (right-side hypertrophy). The right heart will be exhausted much more quickly than the left one. This leads to right heart failure (right heart insufficiency). If the right heart is weak, the blood in the lungs can no longer take in enough oxygen (forward failure), especially since the lungs are usually damaged (chronic pulmonary obstructive disease COPD). In the case of a weak right heart, the blood presses back into the body veins and water enters the tissues of the legs (oedema) and later the body (anasarca).

Cardiac insufficiency is one of the most common internal diseases. It is estimated that about 10 million people in Europe suffer from and are treated for this chronic heart failure. It is estimated that another 10 million have a weak heart that has not yet caused the symptoms of heart failure (compensated cardiac insufficiency). One in 100 among those aged 45 to 55 suffers from cardiac insufficiency, as well as about every tenth person older than 80. A deficit of vitamin D, iron or selenium will facilitate heart muscle weakness. Rare causes include severe anaemia, hyperthyroidism and inflammation of the heart (carditis). Persons suffering from cardiac insufficiency suffer greatly, especially because of shortness of breath (dyspnoea). This often increases when lying down, so that severely affected persons will suffer from threatening night-time fits of shortness of breath and coughing that force them to sleep upright in a reclining chair (orthopnoea).

Cardiac insufficiency usually coincides with other disorders and diseases, such as coronary heart disease, obesity, dyslipidaemia and diabetes. The kidneys are also often affected (renal insufficiency), and anaemia, chronically obstructive pulmonary disease (COPD), muscular atrophy and malnutrition occur frequently. Because of the lack of oxygen in the blood, breathing is often interrupted by long pauses at night (sleep apnoea syndrome), which puts an additional strain on the right heart.

Beginning therapy in time can often successfully tackle cardiac insufficiency, e.g. by implantation of an artificial heart valve or a stent into a constricted coronary vessel. Weight reduction, blood pressure therapy and excretion of water (diuretics) are attempts to relieve the heart. The cardiac output can be improved with digitalis preparations.

Dietary treatment of cardiac insufficiency

Usually patients have already gone through many unsuccessful attempts to lose weight. Weight loss is not possible when the only change is calorie reduction, since overweight persons are hungering for vital substances.

In our experience, fresh fruits and vegetables can save lives specifically for cardiac insufficiency. Here we begin with freshly fruit and vegetable juices prepared with a centrifugal juicer and almond milk (diet stage I). This leads to strong urination (diuresis), so that the oedema (and thus the body weight) and particularly the shortness of breath are quickly and strongly reduced.

Dewatering and detoxing with the fresh juice/almond milk diet will also improve the diabetic metabolism and supply the body with vital substances, secondary plant substances and quantities of highly ordered energy that were missing from the previous nutrition. The care of an experienced doctor is important. Blood values (especially the blood count), creatinine, potassium, sodium, magnesium and selenium must all be monitored. The patients will feel much better within a few weeks. They will be able to breathe more easily and sleep better, and the desired weight reduction and concurrent enrichment with biological energy and vital substances usually returns the heart to a compensated condition. This therapy for cardiac insufficiency is a feasible, scientifically founded[190, 191] and rewarding path for the patient and his doctor. It is a path worth taking.

Heart valve defects

Except for the rare congenital heart valve defects in children, which require surgery at the earliest possible moment, the loss of the sealing of a heart valve (insufficiency) or the occurrence of a narrowing (stenosis) is caused either by inflammation (endocarditis) or by degeneration in the scope of arteriosclerosis.

Mitral valve stenosis

The mitral valve is located in the left heart between the left atrium and left ventricle. Two valve flaps of tough connective tissue are stretched out on tendon strings attached to raised protrusions of heart muscle (papillae) in the left ventricle. During the relaxation phase of the left ventricle (diastole), the latter will be filled with blood by the left atrium through the mitral valve. When ejecting the blood into the aorta, the mitral valve will close tightly to prevent blood from flowing back from the ventricle into the atrium.

Mitral flap stenosis is a narrowing of this valve, so that the blood cannot be pumped from the atrium into the ventricle quickly enough. Mitral flap stenosis is the most commonly acquired heart valve defect in the world. The most common causes are rheumatic fever following an infection of the tonsils (angina) with group A β-haemolysing streptococci. The angina often occurs in a mild form. Afterwards a rheumatic systemic disease in the heart and/or the joints (juvenile rheumatic polyarthritis or Still's disease) will occur, which may also affect the corpus striatum in the brain stem, causing a movement disorder with returning automatisms (Chorea minor, Huntington's disease). Often there will also be ring-shaped reddening of the skin (erythema anulare).

In the heart, rheumatic fever can especially affect the inner layer (endocarditis), the mitral valve and, in about 40 % of cases, the aortic valve simultaneously. The other layers of the heart are also often affected (pancarditis). It still kills about 1–2 out of every 100 affected children and youths, but rarely adults.
Luckily rheumatic carditis has grown rare today, since streptococci can be treated with penicillin. In 50 % of all cases, rheumatic carditis will leave behind chronically rheumatic heart disease. The inflammations leave behind adhesions and scars to the valves, a condition that leads to constriction of the valve openings (stenosis). A bacterial inflammation of the inner layer of the heart, bacterial endocarditis, may also leave behind mitral flap stenosis. Persons with heart valve defects are susceptible to such inflammations of the inner layer of the heart, and they must protect themselves with penicillin in case of infections or dental treatments (endocarditis prophylaxis).

If the opening of the mitral valve is reduced by more than half, this will cause problems for the pulmonary circulation (haemodynamic stenosis), since the blood will be pressed back into the left atrium, which will be overextended by the pressure. This will destroy the conduction pathways in its wall and sooner or later cause atrial fibrillation. The backpressure into the pulmonary veins increases the vascular pressure in the pulmonary circulation, so that pulmonary hypertension occurs which will quickly damage the right heart (pulmonary hypertension).

The valve can sometimes be expanded with a balloon catheter (valvuloplasty). If this is not possible, surgical reconstruction of the valve or valve replacement with an artificial or biological valve must be considered. This can increase life expectancy by approx. 80 %.

Mitral insufficiency

Here the mitral valve between the left atrium and ventricle will not close tightly, so that blood will flow back into the atrium at every heartbeat. This condition is rarely congenital. Like stenosis, mitral insufficiency may be a consequence of rheumatic fever. Usually, however, degenerative changes of the valve in the scope of arteriosclerosis are at fault. It may occur acutely during a posterior myocardial infarction, since one of the valve flaps is attached to the heart muscle. This is a severe condition and usually must be corrected by surgery at once. While congenital diseases of the heart muscle (cardiomyopathies) are rare, congenital mitral valve prolapse is more common. This occurs in persons with connective tissue weakness, in which the flaps are too slack and do not close properly.

Mitral insufficiency is the most common damage to children's hearts in developed countries. To this day, in England and the USA every fiftieth child contracts rheumatic fever. The Framingham study with 3,589 adults showed mitral insufficiency in every fifth person, of equal prevalence in women and men. Eleven percent to 59 % of the patients show mitral insufficiency after a heart attack, while the rate among persons older than 70 with cardiac insufficiency is almost 90 %. In Japan, slight mitral insufficiency is very common.

The normal pressure in the left atrium is 8 mm Hg; that in the ventricle is 120 mm Hg. The pressure increase in the left atrium has a similar effect to that of stenosis, with pulmonary hypertension, expansion of the left atrium, atrial fibrillation, and excessive stress on the right heart up to chronic right heart failure, usually of both ventricles (biventricular cardiac insufficiency).

Medication, chemotherapy and radiation for treating cancer can be further causes. Cytostatics partially damage the heart muscle (e.g. anthracycline, doxorubicin, daunorubicin). The mitral flap is attached to the heart muscle by a tendon. Therefore muscle damage will lead to mitral insufficiency.

A leaking mitral valve makes the patient susceptible to bacterial endocarditis (inflammation of the inner layer of the heart), since bacteria circulating in the blood may settle on the damaged heart valve more easily. Therefore penicillin must be taken for protection in connection with extraction of teeth, any form of suppuration, and for colonoscopies. The doctor will issue an endocarditis pass to ensure prescription of penicillin in such situations.

Surgical therapy corresponds to that for stenosis. Surgical reconstruction of the valve or valve replacement with an artificial or biological valve can be considered. Often an attempt is made to use a cardiac catheter to insert an artificial clamp intended to seal the valve. Surgical interventions come with a relatively high risk, but if successful may considerably improve life expectancy. Persons with only a slight mitral insufficiency have a normal life expectancy. Those with an artificial valve in their hearts usually require permanent anticoagulation treatment (prevention of blood clotting). Blood clots form easily on artificial valves and may be transported to the brain as embolisms (apoplexy).

Aortal valve stenosis

There are congenital forms that must be corrected surgically in childhood. Acquired aortal-valve stenosis results from rheumatic fever after bacterial infection, usually of the tonsils (group A β-haemolysing streptococci), in childhood or youth. Rheumatic carditis will usually damage the mitral valve. This disease has become rare in developed countries. Bacterial infection will lead to acquired aortal stenosis because of bacterial infection of the inner layer of the heart (endocarditis). Patients whose heart valves are already damaged are at increased risk and must carry an endocarditis pass at all times so that they can always be protected with penicillin in time.

Degenerative changes to the valve pockets in connection with arteriosclerosis are by far the most common cause of aortal valve stenosis. Three out of one hundred persons older than 75 suffer from this condition. Valve pockets can adhere and calcify due to degenerative inflammation, similar to that of the vascular walls in arteriosclerosis.
The same risk factors act as a cause. When kidney performance declines (renal insufficiency, raised creatinine), risk increases. The same is true for increased calcium levels in the blood after extended periods of being bedridden or when taking calcium tablets.

It is not rare that someone's aortal valve has only two instead of three valve pockets, a condition that often leads to calcification and constriction (bicuspid aortal valve).

The construction of the aortal valve will lead to more or less of an increased resistance in the left ventricle, depending on the degree of constriction. The left heart is surprisingly adaptable and can thicken its muscle layers (hypertrophy). When the valve narrows down to one fourth of the normal opening size, the heart is no longer able to compensate for the additional stress. This is where left heart failure begins, with reduced blood supply to the head and the entire body (forward failure) and back pressure to the left atrium and the lung The overstressed atrium will extend until atrial fibrillation occurs. The back pressure into the lung causes shortness of breath, up to acute pulmonary oedema, which usually requires emergency admission to the hospital. The back pressure increases the pressure in the pulmonary circulation and damages the right heart until chronic failure of the entire heart results (biventricular cardiac insufficiency).

Severe signs of stress are: shortness of breath when making an effort, angina pectoris and sudden loss of consciousness when making an effort (syncope). The three symptoms are typical for aortal valve stenosis and signify that the survival time – without correction of the aortal valve – is limited to three years.

Slight narrowing of the aortal valve must be monitored annually by a cardiologist using Doppler echocardiography. In some persons the constriction will barely worsen; in others the condition deteriorates more quickly, especially if the valve is already calcified. On average, the valve will narrow by 0.12 cm^2 per year.

Therapeutically, balloon catheter dilatation can be attempted here. Because the valve often narrows again (and quickly), this method should only be considered if surgery is too risky. Surgical replacement with a biological or artificial valve with replacement circulation with the heart-lung machine poses a considerable risk. A minimally invasive valve replacement has become possible for patients in whom the risk in undergoing surgery is too high (TAVI = transcatheter aortic-valve implantation). The artificial valve is pressed into the calcified valve with pressure from a catheter balloon through a catheter inserted through the groin blood vessels or a small cut at the thorax. This can increase a patient's life expectancy somewhat. Permanent anticoagulation therapy will be required after this.

Constriction of the aortic valve will reduce circulation of the coronary vessels. Therefore neither nitro-glycerine, nor blood pressure reducing ACE inhibitors nor calcium antagonists must be taken. At most diuretics can be taken to reduce the circulation volume, but even those must be dosed with care.

Patients with slight aortic stenosis may be normally active. Moderate and most of all severe stenosis requires restraint.

Aortic insufficiency

The causes are the same as those for constriction. There are also rare diseases of the connective tissue. Splitting of the aorta due to progressed arteriosclerosis (aneurysma dissecans) may damage the aortic valve, causing it to leak.

The left heart pushes 40 to 70 ml of blood into the aorta per contraction. If the valve leaks, part of the blood will return to the ventricle during every relaxation phase (diastole). A large difference between the upper (systolic) and lower (diastolic) blood pressure (increased blood pressure amplitude) is common. The blood flowing back puts a volume stress on the left ventricle, which will react by building up muscle (eccentric hypertrophy). Often it can do additional work for many years. If this is not possible anymore, the pressure in the left ventricle will increase at the end of the relaxation phase (end-diastolic pressure). The mitral valve closes prematurely, and chronic left heart failure (left heart insufficiency) will result, as in the case of stenosis and with all the same consequences.

Slight aortic insufficiency must be monitored but does not need to be treated. If the output declines by half or if the patient is suffering shortness of breath, surgical reconstruction of the valve or replacement by an animal or artificial aortic valve should be considered.

Pulmonary valve stenosis

Constrictions of the valve through which the blood is pushed from the right ventricle into the pulmonary artery are usually congenital and rare. Slight constrictions need no therapy. Greater constrictions lead to breathlessness. Physical stress will cause the lips to acquire a bluish tinge (lip cyanosis). The constriction can often be fixed surgically.

Pulmonary valve insufficiency

A slight backflow from the pulmonary artery through the three-part pulmonary valve is common and barely stresses the heart. This is also called "physiological pulmonary valve insufficiency".
Greater leaks often occur due to endocarditis. High pressure in the pulmonary circulation (pulmonary hypertension) will also overextend the pulmonary valve over time, causing it to leak.
Electrocardiography can measure the flow speed of the returning blood and calculate the pressure in the pulmonary artery from this. Dangerous pulmonary

valve insufficiency is much rarer than constriction of this valve.

Tricuspid valve stenosis

The constriction of this valve with three flaps between the right atrium and the right ventricle results from rheumatic fever, usually with damage to the mitral valve. This condition is particularly evident from the back pressure of blood into the vena cava of the systemic circulation. The increased venous pressure in the large circulation due to this causes oedema of the limbs and the abdominal cavity (ascites). This valve defect can be removed by surgical opening (valvulotomy) or an artificial heart valve.

Tricuspid valve insufficiency

The cause is usually a pulmonary embolism or increased pressure in the pulmonary artery due to lung disease. Leaking of the three flaps causes backflow of blood from the right ventricle into the right atrium.

Electrocardiography will reveal slight leaks in up to 89 % of all adults, especially in athletes who train to the point of hypertrophy. The leaks are usually harmless (physiological insufficiency). More severe forms of tricuspid valve insufficiency are rarely congenital and usually appear with other heart defects. Acquired leaks result from overexpansion of the valve ring due to pulmonary hypertension or may be acute because of pulmonary embolism. If a clot gets into a large pulmonary vessel, the pressure in the pulmonary artery is increased massively at once. The valve will leak immediately.

Tricuspid valve insufficiency is a relatively common valve defect. Precise figures are not known. More than 60 cm^3 of blood flowing between the right ventricle and right atrium is considered severe. If this happens acutely, there may be potentially fatal disorders. The pressure in the vena cava increases to 50 mm Hg and causes acute venous congestion in the liver, the carotid veins and all body veins. When the acute stage is past, or if the insufficiency develops slowly, the atrium first enlarges, often to three or four times its size and the right ventricle develops more muscle (hypertrophy). The lung does not receive enough blood (breathlessness) and the increased pressure in the body veins causes water to enter the tissues (oedemas). Over time the right ventricle expands more and more, expanding the valve ring even further, causing valve insufficiency to increase dramatically.

Slight forms remain unnoticed, but severe forms become evident through oedema, carotid vein congestion, liver congestion and often through skipped heartbeats (extrasystoles) or racing heart (tachycardia).
Severe forms often remain stable for a long time, as long as they do not overload the right ventricle. This condition must be monitored regularly. The patients need endocarditis prophylaxis with penicillin, since they are at high risk. If the right atrium is considerably enlarged, anticoagulation is necessary to prevent the danger of pulmonary embolism. Surgical restoration by valve reconstruction or replacement with an artificial valve is rather rarely recommended, especially where due to the chronic liver congestion, which may lead to liver cirrhosis, or where the condition as such may become threatening.

Inflammatory diseases of the heart

Myocarditis

Many cases of myocarditis from viral infections go unnoticed. However, there may also be potentially fatal arrhythmia, up to death from ventricular fibrillation. When all three layers of the heart are affected, the condition is called pancarditis.

In the USA it is estimated that 1 % to 5 % of all viral infections attack the heart. The frequency of myocarditis is estimated at approx. 5 per 100,000 residents per year.

More than half of the cases of myocarditis in Europe and the USA are caused by enteroviruses. This group of echo- and coxsackie viruses (B1-5) causes summer flu with diarrhoea and a typical two-peaked fever. Apart from this, parvovirus B 19, adenoviruses, influenza viruses and mumps viruses could be isolated from the heart muscle.

Cases of myocarditis from bacteria almost always occur in persons with impaired immune systems (HIV, immunosuppressive therapy). The germs are brucelles, pneumococci and the pathogens for diphtheria and tuberculosis. In South America, the Chagas disease and the single-cell organism Trypanosoma cruzi can attack the heart, while in Canada fungi (aspergillus) must be monitored.

In Europe, Lyme disease from tick bites may attack the heart, and more rarely leptospires and rickettsias. Carditis can be transferred from mother to child, though occurrences are rare.

Toxic myocardial damage

Poisoning may also cause myocarditis The most common form is alcohol, while heavy metal poisoning is rarer. Poisoning of the heart muscle due to chemotherapy against cancer (anthracyclines, cyclophosphamide, fluorouracil) is not uncommon. Barbiturates to treat epilepsy and a number of psychotropic drugs are also toxic to the heart.

Autoimmune inflammation of the heart

Some autoimmune diseases attack the heart. The most dangerous ones are vasculitis (autoallergic vascular inflammation throughout the body), sarcoidose (Boeck's disease), systemic Lupus erythematodes and sclerodermia.

The symptoms of myocarditis, treatment and prognosis

Myocarditis will most often become evident from fatigue, fever, palpitations of the heart, shortness of breath and a general feeling of being unwell. Cardiac arrest due to ventricular fibrillation is rare. Treatment of viruses with interferons is not yet fully established.

In most cases, myocarditis will heal spontaneously without subsequent problems. Toxic myocarditis has a chronic progression, often requiring medication against heart failure.

Endocarditis

Disease of the inner layer of the heart affects the heart cavities, the heart valves, and the inner layers of the large arteries and veins close to the heart. It may affect anyone but will occur particularly in those whose heart valves are already damaged. Untreated it is fatal in most cases.

Treatment with antibiotics has changed the prognosis, and the disease has become rare in Western Europe. However, infections with very bad prognosis from multi-resistant bacteria found in hospitals and nursing homes (nosocomial infections) are more common today.

Aneurysm

An aneurysm is a localised bulge of an arterial wall.
Congenital weaknesses of the wall are rare. Inflammations or injuries of the arterial wall may leave an aneurysm. Usually, however, it is produced by arteriosclerosis. Men over 50 are often affected. Most of them are patients with hypertension or arteriosclerosis in the leg arteries (peripheral vascular disease PVD). Tears in an arteriosclerosis plaque that pass through the entire wall of the vessel will cause a bulge in it due to the pulsating pressure (aneurysm). A defect that tears it open further may be life threatening.

Aneurysm dissecans of the aorta

The aneurysma dissecans of the aorta is a very dangerous form of rupture of an arterial wall. The damage often remains concealed at first, while the strong aortal wall is splitting in length through its layers because of the high pulsating pressure of the blood (dissection). This produces a second pulsating vascular lumen that will burst open into the inner thorax or the abdominal cavity at some point and is fatal.

If a dissecting aortic aneurysm reaches a diameter of 50 mm in the ultrasound examination, surgery is urgently required.

Aneurysms of the cerebral arteries

Small cerebral aneurysms of the arteries in the brain will be monitored to see if they enlarge. Large aneurysms must be treated because of the danger of cerebral haemorrhage. There is also the option of endovascular therapy, with which a catheter makes it possible to reach up to the aneurysm where a platinum coil is inserted into the aneurysm sac. This coil produces a firmly attached blood clot, so that the blood is no longer pressed into the aneurysm sac with its high pulsation pressure. Sometimes a stent is also introduced into the aneurysm, with the hope that the arterial wall will be stabilised.

Open surgery of the aneurysm requires opening of the skull and open access to the aneurysm. The aneurysm sac is then closed with a clamp. Neurological damage cannot always be avoided during this surgery.

Stroke (apoplexy)

A stroke is one of the worst disasters that a person can experience. It is a typical consequence of arteriosclerosis. A stroke is also called a CVA (cerebrovascular accident).

There are different causes of stroke: occlusion of a vessel (ischaemic stroke), acute cerebral haemorrhage (haemorrhagic stroke), and the bursting of an arterial expansion (aneurysm haemorrhage). Primarily ischaemic cerebral infarction may also lead to subsequent bleeding that will destroy cerebral tissue.

In Germany, each year about 200 out of every 100,000 persons suffer an ischaemic stroke, i.e. one out of 500. In addition to this, there are 24 aneurysm haemorrhages among 100,000 persons, 6 strokes among 100,000 inhabitants due to acute bleeding from a vessel into the brain fluid (subarachnoid haemorrhage), and 8 apoplexies for undetermined reasons. At one stroke per 420 persons per year, apoplexy is one of the most common diagnoses, and the third most common cause of death (approx. 65,000 deaths per year). In addition to this, there is the suffering with often most severe physical and mental disability among those who survive an apoplexy.

In case of sudden paralysis or clouding of consciousness, the doctor will immediately have an examination performed by computer tomography (CT) or magnetic resonance tomography (MR). Blood dilution must be discontinued immediately to prevent further haemorrhage.
Sometimes the symptoms can be very minor and recede again without 24 hours (this used to be aptly called a transient ischaemic attack (TIA). A subarachnoid haemorrhage from very small vessels may only produce a headache and can be confirmed by a careful spinal tap. In contrast, larger ones are acutely life threatening, with a sudden loss of consciousness due to pressure on the brain and threatening cardiovascular arrest.

Typical symptoms are: one- or two-sided visual impairment, double images or loss of the field of vision, loss of perception of part of the environment or one's own body (neglect), vertigo, nausea, vomiting, gait disorder, balance or coordination problems (ataxia), numbness, paralysis or weakness in the face, an arm, leg or the entire side of the body, confusion, disorientation, comprehensive and speech impairment, aphasia, distorted writing, severe headache without recognisable cause, possibly with increased blood pressure, and difficulty in swallowing (dysphagia).

Common causes of apoplexy are: embolism of the brain due to passage of a blood clot at atrial fibrillation, bursting of an arteriosclerotically changed arterial wall during a blood pressure crisis, haemorrhage from an extreme anticoagulation or massive cramping of an arteriosclerotic vessel during a migraine attack. Persons in danger of falling must only be given very slight anticoagulation, or inhibition of the adhesion capacities of the blood platelets (thrombocyte aggregation inhibition), since such persons would be in great danger of haemorrhage if they fell on their head.

An immediate emergency call for admission to hospital is decisive for prognosis, since thrombolyse therapy, where possible, must be started within 3–4 hours. Until then the upper body should be raised, and the patient must not be given food or drink, since there is danger of the patient's choking, leading to dangerous pneumonia. Any physical effort must be avoided until the patient is taken to an emergency room of an acute hospital or a specialised stroke unit by ambulance.

Often it is possible to dissolve the blood clot by thrombolytic medication to partially save brain tissue. In more than 60 % of the patients with an occlusion of a large brain artery, it is possible to save enough brain tissue after immediate removal of the blood clot with a catheter (neurothrombectomy) for them to be able to lead an acceptable independent life again after only three months of rehabilitation. However, this procedure can only be applied in about 15 % of the patients with stroke. If there is no atrial fibrillation, a long-term electrocardiogram (Holter) for 72 hours is required to determine if there is temporary atrial fibrillation as a cause (intermittent atrial fibrillation). After the acute phase, permanent anticoagulation is usually required.

Neuro-rehabilitation requires great commitment and empathy, as well as a lot of patience and cooperation on the part of both patient and therapists. Perception, new gait and movement patterns must be practised with a physical therapist. The scarring region of the brain will functionally impair adjacent areas as well. Therefore, transcranial magnetic stimulation (through the skull) may improve the mobility of a paralysed limb. In this sense the acupuncture of the skull according to Yamamoto as introduced in a large rehabilitation clinic in Japan or stimulation of affected brain regions by neural therapy also brings good results. Homoeopathy can limit the damage in the acute phase by approx. hourly administration of arnica montana in the hundred-thousandth potency, and during the rehabilitation phase by administration of hypericum several times a day in the same potency.

The disaster of apoplexy can be prevented. The decisive and most reasonable therapy is prevention. It is sensible to start this even in childhood. This book gives attentive readers everything they need to know and the practical instruction for it. Observing these recommendations will reliably prevent such disasters.

Renal artery stenosis

The most frequent cause of constriction of the renal artery is arteriosclerosis. More rarely, a connective tissue disorder in the vessel may cause renal artery stenosis in young adults. Rare causes are autoimmune inflammation of the artery (arteritis), injury or thrombosis.

The kidney that has lost sufficient circulation will produce the hormone renin without interruption, since it is getting too little blood. This will lead to dangerous high blood pressure (malignant hypertension).

In 80 % of the cases, the constriction can be removed by catheter dilatation (percutaneous transluminal angioplasty, or PTA). If this is not possible, the kidney must be supplied with a bypass vessel in open surgery.

Carotid artery stenosis

This constriction of a large cerebral artery (Arteria carotis communis or Arteria carotis interna) usually results from arteriosclerosis. Only rarely is it caused by an autoimmune inflammation (vasculitis).

The carotid artery stenosis can exist without symptoms for a long time. Ultimately, however, there will be volatile small brain infarctions (transient ischaemic attacks), which are seen as precursors of a larger brain infarction, or volatile loss of vision (amaurosis fugax) if the central retinal artery is occluded temporarily. Such precursors must be taken very seriously. Ninety percent of brain infarctions (apoplexies) happen in the carotid arteries.

Every year in Germany approx. 30,000 persons suffer an apoplexy because of arteriosclerotic constrictions in the carotid arteries.

When the cerebral artery is constricted by less than 80 %, there are no symptoms and the annual apoplexy risk is at 1–2 %. When both carotid arteries are constricted, the risk is much higher.
The carotid artery stenosis may be reversed by the diet suggested by this book and heal slowly in the course of many months.
If there already are symptoms, catheter dilatation or surgical opening (endarterectomy) must be considered.

Peripheral vascular disease (PVD)

Arteriosclerotic constrictions in leg arteries, and rarely the aorta, prevent the blood supply from flowing to the extremities. After varying walking distances, there will be a lack of oxygen and cramping pain that forces the affected person to stop. This is called claudicatio intermittens or intermittent claudication. Four and a half million people in Germany suffer from this disease. If an artery closes all the way where there is no bypass circulation available, the affected area of the leg will die (gangrene).

Such vascular occlusions are often treated surgically by opening the inside of the artery (endarterectomy) or inserting a piece of vein as a bypass.

The diet as described in this book and daily gait training may slowly reduce the constriction of the leg artery. The patient will be rewarded by a slow but steady extension of the possible walking distance before uninhibited walking and hiking can be resumed.

Arrhythmia

Interferences of the heart rhythm (arrhythmia) mean an impairment of the regular sequence of heartbeats.
The muscles of the heart are designed very differently from those in the body, in that the membranes of the muscle cells continually discharge on their own until this causes the muscle fibres to contract, upon which the membrane potential will be built up again. Special muscle fibres (Purkinje fibres) form centres of excitation formation and the conduction pathway system of the heart. It originates in the sinus node in the right atrium. From there, the fibres run to a second node between the left atrium and the ventricle, the AV-node; inside the ventricles, they spread towards the bottom and the tip of the heart with a certain amount of branching.

Domination takes place from the top down. In a healthy heart, the sinus node with its regular rhythm will always forestall the slower fibres because its discharges come earlier than those of the AV-node. The AV-node on its own would only discharge the ventricles at a slower rhythm of barely 40 beats per minute.

The normal healthy rhythm of the heart is called a sinus rhythm. It initially excites contraction of the atria and very quickly after that the ventricles via the AV-node. This sequence is reflected in the electrocardiogram, by the small p-wave of the atrial contraction and the subsequent QRS-peak of the ventricular discharge, followed after a moment by a T-wave, which is caused by the recharging of the ventricular muscles (repolarisation).

The sinus node is stimulated to work at a faster and stronger rhythm by excitation of the sympathetic nervous system and the adrenal hormone adrenaline. The parasympathetic nervous system, as opponent, slows the rhythm and weakens it, to make the heart come to rest. The thyroid hormone thyroxin, in contrast, accelerates the rhythm by driving the metabolism in the sense of combustion and consumption throughout the body. Thus, the rhythm is too fast at hyperthyrosis and is too slow at hypothyrosis.

Disorders of the heart rhythm occur when the healthy sequence in the conduction pathway system is impaired, e.g. by overexpansion of the heart, lack of oxygen in the muscles due to arteriosclerotic changes in the coronary vessels (coronary sclerosis) or diseases of the heart muscle due to hyperthyrosis or other metabolic disorders or disorders of the electrolyte balance. Congenital malformations of the conduction pathway system are rare.

A pathologically slow rhythm is called bradycardia, one that is too fast is called tachycardia. Accordingly, there are bradycard and tachycard arrhythmias. The arrhythmias are usually named after the place of origin in the conduction pathway system. Consequently, they may be harmless or very dangerous.

Supraventricular extrasystoles

The left atrium may initiate additional beats if a place below the sinus node forestalls it. These are usually harmless.

Often the extra beats are not noticed, or are noticed only as a small skip. It is the compensating pause, rather than the early beat, that will be noticed.

A disease of the heart, a cardiovascular disease, a thyroid or electrolyte disorder must be ruled out. Then this disorder can often be corrected by a professionally chosen homoeopathic therapy or neural therapy of the heart's sympathetic nervous system.

Ventricular extrasystoles

These extra beats are produced in the ventricle. They become dangerous when occurring in volleys, where they may be precursors of cardiac arrest because of ventricular fibrillation.

Atrial flutter and atrial fibrillation (absolute arrhythmia)

About six million persons in Europe suffer from atrial fibrillation, i.e. about every seventieth European. Numbers increase with age: 0.5 % of those under 40 years old, but up to 15 % of those aged over 80. Men are affected more often than women. The costs caused by atrial fibrillation for EU-countries are estimated at 13.5 billion euros. The number of hospital stays due to atrial fibrillation has increased by 66 % over the past decade. Mortality from atrial fibrillation is about twice that of persons of the same age with a normal heart rhythm. On average, about 6 % of the persons with atrial fibrillation will suffer a stroke. 15–20 % of all strokes happen from atrial fibrillation. This reduces life expectancy by 25 %.

Intermittent atrial fibrillation goes unnoticed by the patient in 70 % of all cases (fibrillation attacks). If the fibrillation persists, however, sudden performance drops, and fatigue, palpitations or new sleeping problems will cause patients to see their general practitioner.

Causes of atrial fibrillation

Atrial fibrillation may occur without recognisable cause (idiopathic lone atrial fibrillation), as is the case in 45 % of intermittent and 25 % of permanent atrial fibrillations. About 25 % suffer from arterial occlusive disease due to arteriosclerosis and another 25 % from hypertension, 20 % from a heart valve defect and about 15 % from myocarditis. Atrial fibrillation is found in 40 % of all patients with chronic heart failure (cardiac insufficiency). In about 2 % of the same population hyperthyrosis occurs and the risk of this impairment increases fivefold. Surgical interventions with opening of the chest cavity may trigger atrial fibrillation. Congenital causes are rare. Excessive training for competitive sports may also facilitate atrial fibrillation.

Persistent hypertension will overextend the left atrium, which will damage the excitation pathway system. The discharges in the atrial muscles can no longer be controlled by the sinus node and there are often quick circular excitations of the muscle fibres in the pulmonary veins close to the heart, causing the atria to contract only uncoordinatedly and in a weakly fluttering or fibrillating manner. Once the fibrillation is present, the atria will deform and the calcium flow into the muscle cells will become reduced, so that fibrillation cannot disappear again easily.

The ventricles will then discharge in a very irregular rhythm (absolute arrhythmia), usually at a rhythm that is too fast (tachycard atrial fibrillation) and the output of the heart by approx. 15 %.

Alcohol and atrial fibrillation

This atrial fibrillation called Holiday Heart Syndrome typically occurs a few hours after excessive alcohol intake. It will usually end again within 24 hours. Nevertheless, the Danish Diet Cancer and Health Study showed that the risk for permanent atrial fibrillation for men and women consuming more than 12 g of pure alcohol per day was almost twice as high; and for men starting at a consumption of more than 20 g of pure alcohol per day, the study even documented a 44 % risk increase.

Risk of embolism
Atrial fibrillation is dangerous because the uncontrolled blood flow in the atrium may cause blood clots (thrombi) to form, which may pass to the brain (embolism of the brain, brain infarction, apoplexy). These thrombi usually occur in a kind of pocket, the auricle. Mesenterial embolisms are rarer. In this case, a blood clot enters an intestinal artery.

Anticoagulation (inhibition of blood clotting)
The risk of embolism can be clearly reduced by anticoagulation, usually by inhibiting the adhesiveness of the blood platelets (thrombocyte aggregation inhibition) with amino salicylic acid (ASS) or to a greater extent with coumarins, which are taken as tablets but require monitoring of the coagulation. As an alternative, new platelet aggregation inhibitors are available (NOAC = new oral anti-coagulants), such as Dabigatranetexilat, Rivaroxaban or Apixaban and others. As compared to coumarins, these new medicines reduce the embolism risk to the same extent, but with a lower risk of haemorrhage. The danger of haemorrhage, both spontaneous and in case of injuries, is the problem with anticoagulation. This risk of haemorrhage increases only slightly with age, while the embolism risk increases by 1.4 % per ten years of additional age. If embolisms have already occurred, the risk increases by 2.5 %, hypertension will increase it by 1.6 %, and diabetes by 1.7 %. If the embolism risk is very high, an attempt can be made to insert a catheter to close the auricle so that fewer thrombi can form.

The type of anticoagulation must be chosen with great care by the doctor. A CHA_2DS_2VASC score specifies globally valid guidelines for this. The European Society of Cardiology has issued a HAS-BLED score to estimate the risk of cerebral haemorrhage.

Tachycard atrial fibrillation
Tachycardia will reduce the heart's output significantly. Beta-blockers, digitalis, diltiazem or verapamil can slow the tachycardia to a frequency of 60 to 80 beats per minute, so that the heart output will improve. If the rhythm is slowed too much (under 50 beats per minute), there is a risk of dangerous loss of consciousness (syncopes), which may cause severe head injuries and cerebral haemorrhage since a fall cannot be excluded.

An increased rhythm amplitude is present when the absolute arrhythmia has very early and very late beats, leading to further reduction of the output. This may be promptly and clearly improved by neural therapy stimulation of the sympathetic nervous system of the heart.

Cardioversion
An atrial fibrillation once first discovered often spontaneously ends again within 24 hours. If it persists, it can often be returned to the normal sinus rhythm by electro conversion. Under brief anaesthesia, a device that reads the electrocardiogram is used to administer an automatically controlled electrical shock to the heart, as during reanimation, but at a lower dose. Antiarrhythmics are often administered then, such as Amiodaron, Flecainid or beta blockers.

Catheter ablation
If the fibrillation returns, catheter ablation may help. The heart catheter is used

to place longitudinal injuries of the inner layer of the heart (endocardium) of the left atrium, or muscle bundles at the entries of the pulmonary veins are removed in rings (pulmonary vein isolation), to remove the interference coming from the pulmonary veins. In about 65 % of patients, this intervention improves the condition, but such interventions are difficult, time consuming and come with a relatively high risk of embolism as well as the risk that the pulmonary veins will constrict too much afterwards (pulmonary vein stenosis). The method of improving fibrillation by pacemaker therapy is still in the trial stage.

Tachycardia

A heart frequency above 100 beats per minute is called tachycardia. This is a normal performance adjustment of the heart to physical stress. Toddlers have an equally high pulse, even at rest.

If the fast pulse starts suddenly without physical effort, this is called *paroxysmal tachycardia*.
In adults, tachycardia above 120 beats per minute may be dangerous. From 150 beats per minute onwards, immediate treatment is required. Such a frequency at rest will reduce available energy.

High fever, fear and panic, electrolyte disorders or massive blood loss will produce a fast heart frequency that originates in the sinus node *(Birchermuesli)*.

In the *Birchermuesli*, the atrium triggers the tachycardia. The ventricle will not take over all heartbeats (pulse deficit). The electrocardiogram serves diagnostic purposes. Here, a point in the conduction pathway system of the atrium will produce tachycardia.

If the excitation circulates between the atrium and ventricle, it is called an AV-Reentry tachycardia. This appears suddenly. The cause is a congenital additional pathway that creates a short circuit between the ventricle and the atrium. As an emergency therapy, adenosine is injected intravenously. It blocks the transmission in the atrium temporarily (AV-block III).

Attempts are made to heal this disorder with electrical heart frequency controlled sclerotherapy of the accessory pathway by heart catheter. Beta blockers and calcium antagonists slow the transmission in the atrium and sometimes reduce the frequency of such attacks. The antiarrhythmics Flecainid or Propafenon may also be tried.

A double formation of the AV-node between the atrium and ventricle may cause benign attacks of tachycardia (AV-nodal reentry tachycardia).

Wolff-Parkinson White syndrome, a congenital anomaly of the conduction pathway system, produces paroxysmal tachycardia at frequencies of 150–220 contractions per minute together with great weakness. The attack can often be interrupted by drinking iced water, by pushing on the carotid artery or through injection of antiarrhythmics under hospital conditions. If this is not possible, an electro-conversion under short anaesthesia is required, as in the case of tachycard atrial fibrillation.

Transmission impairment in the tracks of the atria (bundle branch block) may also cause arrhythmias in strong blocks, where the ventricle will no longer be excited by every action of the heart (2:1 block). This disorder can also often be eliminated by neural therapy of the sympathetic nervous system of the heart.

Ventricular tachycardia is evident at once in the ECG. The disorder originates in the ventricle. This form of tachycardia is a very dangerous precursor of cardiac arrest from ventricular fibrillation. As in the case of cardiac arrest by ventricular fibrillation, defibrillation is required.

Inflammation of the arteries

Arteries are mostly inflamed in the case of autoimmune diseases.

Vasculitis

Vasculitis means inflammation of the vessels caused by autoimmune diseases (type III allergy). The inflammation may affect all vessels, arteries, the smaller arterioles, the capillary system, the veins, and thus also damage many organs. Vasculitis is dangerous. It used to kill within weeks or months. Today the acute destructive effects can be suppressed by immunosuppression to protect organs in the acute phase. However, this does not remove the massive loss of control of the immune systems, which has forgotten how to distinguish external from internal.
The cause of vasculitis is considered to be unknown. Genetic factors, infections with the bacterium staphylococcus aureus or hepatitis viruses are sometimes mentioned as possible causes.

If there is no underlying disease, the inflammation is called *primary vasculitis*. Types of vasculitides are classified according to the size of the affected vessels and by whether the ANCA antibodies are found or not.

Vasculitides with ANCA antibodies
Granulomatosis with polyangiitis (formerly Wegener granulomatosis)
This autoimmune vasculitis is rare. It affects persons in middle age; women are at higher risk. Children are rarely affected. Vessels in the nasopharyngeal cavity and the lungs, and in later stages the small vessels of the kidneys, will be damaged.

The eosinophil granulomatosis with polyangiitis (formerly Churg-Strauss syndrome)
This vasculitis is caused by IgE antibodies and produces grains (granulomas) in the vessels. It starts with an allergic cold, then a cough, asthma and allergic intestinal inflammation. It may affect the blood vessels of other organs later.

Microscopic polyarteritis (MPA, mPAN)
This disease is very rare and attacks vessels in the skin, the kidneys, the lung, and at later stages the eyes, nervous system and all organs.

Vasculitides without ANCA antibodies
Here, the smallest vessels will have deposits of antigen-antibody complexes, called immune-complexes, and also protein deposits (complement) from the unspecific immune system that is not directed against specific allergy-triggering causes. This includes:

IgA-vasculitis (Purpura Schönlein-Henoch)
This form of vasculitis of the smallest vessels affects approx. 5 out of 1,000 children and youths. It mostly affects the vessels of the skin and in various organs, especially the kidneys. It is often caused by infection or medication.

Vasculitis with cryoglobulinaemia
This is an inflammation of smallest vessels that is caused by the effect of cold.

Cutaneous leucocytoclastic angiitis
This is a vascular inflammation where immune complexes attack the smallest vessels, especially in the skin.

Primary vasculitides of medium-sized vessels
This self-destructive vascular inflammation occurs without underlying disease and attacks medium-sized vessels.

Polyarteritis nodosa (PAN or cPAN)
This autoimmune disease attacks medium-sized vessels in all organs and damages all organs, including the nervous system, the skin and the kidneys. It sometimes appears like an inflammation of the liver (hepatitis B). It is called nodosa because it forms nodules.

Kawasaki syndrome
This is an auto-allergic inflammation of medium-sized vessels in many organs that particularly affects toddlers and initially looks similar to measles. The auto-allergic inflammation destroys small and medium-sized vessels. It is suspected that genetic causes and infections can trigger this syndrome.

Primary vasculitides of large vessels
These auto-allergic inflammations attack large vessels.

Giant-cell arteritis Norton (Arteritis temporalis, Arteritis cranialis)
Without an underlying disease, a dangerous auto-allergic inflammation appears, particularly in the temporal arteries of older persons, especially women. Without treatment, 20 % of the patients will go blind, since the circulation of the retina is endangered.

Takayasu arteritis
Without underlying disease, an auto-allergic inflammation rarely appears in young women's aortas and their main branches. There are no ANCA-antibodies. Takayasu arteritis causes fever and general symptoms of illness, and often produces hypertension with the risk of stroke.

Secondary arteritides
These are auto-allergic inflammations of the vessels, in connection with general auto-allergic underlying disease or infections, such as AIDS or syphilis. This also includes acute rejection reactions of the immune systems against a transplanted organ. Cocaine or ergot alkaloids (ergotamine) and specific healing herbs (rare) may also cause auto-allergic vascular inflammation.

Unclassifiable arteritides
Endangiitis obliterans
Autoallergic inflammation results from the pollutants of smoking, particularly in middle-aged men, and attacks arteries and veins of the extremities.

Behcet syndrome
This auto-immune disease affects mostly men from Turkey and the Middle East, starting in middle age. Genetic causes are suspected. Infections may trigger episodes. It is assigned to the rheumatic circle. The inflammations come in episodes and attack the mucosa of the mouth and the sexual organs, as well as almost all structures in the eyes, heightening the risk of blindness.

Cerebral vasculitis
Very rarely younger persons develop an autoimmune inflammation of the cerebral vessels without an underlying disease, or in the context of a general vasculitis. It may be triggered by infections. Headache, paralysis or sensation impairment, and behavioural changes are similar to the symptoms of a stroke.

Treatment of vasculitides
These auto-immune inflammations are very dangerous. Depending on the organs

that the affected vessels supply, there is a great danger of their very considerable destruction to a large extent and the effect on the lives of the persons affected. Therefore cortisol and, if necessary, other immune-suppressants must be administered as emergency intervention in an acute episode, to suppress the uncontrolled hyperactivity of the immune system.

The emergency therapy protects the vessels and saves the organs but will not heal the massive derailment of the immune system, which has forgotten how to distinguish between what is foreign and what is its own, and thus vehemently attacks the body's own structures.

The immune cells are formed in the bone marrow. The lymphocytes wander into the billions of lymph follicles of the intestinal mucosa. Inside the intestine, the enormous surface of the sensitive mucosa continually comes into contact with foreign substances. In the immune system of the intestine, the lymphocytes learn their immune competence, i.e. to differentiate between what is foreign and what is its own. Only 10 % of them acquire this ability and then move on to the lymph nodes throughout the body (and into the vessels) to perform their relevant tasks.

If the milieu inside the intestine is impaired by widespread poor nutrition, the bacterial flora is often massively impaired and the mucosa irritated. In a healthy person, the intestinal mucosa is covered by a thick mucus layer that contains an entire "catalogue" of IgA antibodies that are there so as to tell the immune cells what belongs and what does not, and which foreign substances are permitted in the intestine, since they are known not to harm the body. The lymphocytes learn their immune-competence here.

In our experience, consistent elimination of this problem is critical for the healing of any auto-immune disease. Auto-immune diseases are not healed by medication, but slowly and over many months with a vegetarian raw food diet allergologically adapted to the patient by IgG4 testing, which will keep the patients from further destruction and risks to their lives. This initially often requires in-patient therapy with careful medical checks and support. It is a path that is worth the effort.

The diseases and therapy of the venous system are treated in the Bircher-Benner manual no. 13: *Manual for venous diseases*.

Regulative treatments of naturopathic healing for cardiovascular patients

Climate therapy and terrain treatments

The bracing climates of the high mountains and by the North Sea are too strong for persons with hypertension and heart disease. Low mountain ranges and the Baltic Sea are ideal for holidays or spa treatments. It is often difficult to get the right diet in hotels and spa houses, since they often cook too generously in order to please their guests.

Those unable to hike because of severe heart failure will slowly regain their strength by lying in the fresh air for several hours every day (lying treatment). Those who can walk or hike should hike by the sea or uphill at a moderate inclination dressed in coolish clothes, starting with one hour per day and increasing the duration every day, but keeping to a leisurely pace. The physical performance will improve noticeably every day.

Hydrotherapy

This is a very valuable and highly effective regulation therapy that you can apply yourself. It is important that you should be thoroughly warm before beginning any cold treatment. Particularly at the beginning, you should start with a short cold water stimulus that is not too strong, and slowly increase this day by day. Warm treatments produce passive warmth to which the body reacts by cooling off. Cold treatments produce active heat as counter-regulation to the cooling. It has a much greater regulative effect than passive warming.

Cold body compress

Once a week, a cold body compress in the evening may help reduce blood pressure. Place a plastic sheet on a bed covered with a woollen blanket. Fold a linen cloth so that it will reach from the pelvis to below the armpits, wet it with cold water, wring it out and place it across the woollen blanket. While lying down on it. inhale deeply, fold it tightly around you and fold the woollen blanket over it, then cover yourself with a warm duvet. The body compress will lead to a deep internal warming, increase the nightly reducing of circulation, and lower blood pressure. It can be left on for 2 to 5 hours.

The thigh gush

First thing in the morning every day. In the shower, sitting on a stool, after thoroughly warming yourslf, pour cold water on your feet, lower legs and thighs. Then rest while covered up. Produces deep inner warmth, improves thermal regulation and circulatory regulation of the body, increasing internal stability.

Treading water

Thrice a week, in the later afternoon or evening. Place a large plastic tub in the shower, fill it with cold water to approx. 25 cm and tread in it for about 5 minutes. Rest covered up. Water treading will withdraw accumulated energy from the head, release pointless repetitive thoughts, and thus make it easier to fall asleep.

Alternating foot bath

Twice a week in the late afternoon or early evening. Prepare a large bucket container of very hot water and a second one of very cold water. Start in the hot water until you are well warmed, then switch to cold water, stay there for 2 minutes, then return to hot water until well warmed, and then back into cold water for 1 minute. Dry off and rest well covered up. The alternating foot bath stabilises circulation and considerably promotes regulation and thermal regulation. It calms pointless repetitive thoughts and makes it easier to fall asleep.

Rising arm bath

Twice a week. Fill a washbasin with warm water, immerse your arms to the middle of the upper arm, slowly increase the temperature to 42–45 degrees. Keep doing this for 10 minutes, until you start to sweat, then briefly wash your arms with a washcloth and rest covered up.
Rising foot bath with the same procedure, or both at the same time with a helper. This is passive heating that will withdraw energy accumulated in the head and will often also help alleviate headaches. The brief cold washing in the end triggers active regulation.

Neck gush

Daily when a melancholy mood occurs. After warming up thoroughly, sit in the shower, bend forward a little and pour cold water onto your neck, upper back and sternum. Start with a short duration, increase over time. In the case of drowsiness, fatigue, apply a short, cold gush to the top of the head and the face. Invigorates mind and spirit, brightens the mood. The top of the head has important reflex zones of the brain stem ganglia and the limbic system that are stimulated by this.

Classical homoeopathic treatment

Homeopathy is based on the experiences of Samuel Hahnemann that certain physical procedures permit the release of immaterial medicinal effects from matter. By means of step-by-step dilution and considerable mechanical shaking, specific information from the original substance is saved in the energetic structure of the alcohol molecule or sugar molecule and made durable.

Homeopathy is pure information therapy. Homeopathic medication is comparable to a kind of programme disc that – similar to computer technology – permits entering ordering information into the human organism. The homeopathic medicinal effect is not material, i.e. it does not directly manipulate the biochemical processes as a molecule or substance, but in a higher way, as an ordering impulse on an electromagnetic path. This is where the ingenious minds of Maximilian Bircher-Benner and Samuel Hahnemann meet. Bircher-Benner researched the non-material ordering effect of fresh raw fruit and vegetable food on chronic diseases in decades of clinical work, while Hahnemann released non-material ordering information from substances and observed their effects on the healthy and finally the sick human.

The homeopathic medicinal effect is highly specific. The only medication capable of providing the healing (ordering) impulse is that which provokes exactly the same symptoms in the healthy person as those that are to be healed in the ill person. Therefore a precise collecting of symptoms and a basic understanding of the personality and current mood of the patient are an absolute prerequisite for finding the right medication.

Homoeopathy alone cannot heal cardiovascular diseases. The diet and new order of life described in this book are decisive for this. Sometimes it is possible to influence certain emotional causes of hypertension and certain arrhythmias very positively, even those that have withstood many years of psychotherapy. In practical experience, nitroglycerine in the thousandth potency (Glonoinum MK) has proved to be as effective in stable angina pectoris as unpotentiated medicine, with the benefit of few adverse side effects such as hot flushes and headache. The treatment can be repeated several times at short intervals. Nevertheless, patients will have to have unpotentiated nitroglycerine on their persons at all times and use it at once if the Glonoinum does not immediately remove the pain. If this does not work immediately either, the patient may be suffering a heart attack and an emergency doctor must be informed at once. Homoeopathic high potency digitalis may also be helpful for certain arrhythmias. In any case, homoeopathic therapy belongs in the hands of a doctor or a healer well experienced in classical homoeopathy and who works closely with the attending physician.

The new scientific acupuncture

Acupuncture is one of the oldest methods for stimulating and guiding the regulation activity of the organism.

In the last few years, it has already received a fairly solid scientific basis, as can be seen in many examples of basic research.[192] Benifiting from its thousands of years of research into therapeutic effects, Chinese medicine has shown how the individual organs, muscle groups and body layers are interconnected. These ancient scientific conclusions are in agreement with the latest scientific findings on the vegetative nervous system and the basic regulation system of the soft connective tissue. According to Chinese medicine (TCM), outer (e.g. climate and seasonable) influences and inner factors such as stress on the mind may cause our basic regulation to lose its manifold balance, and thus bring on diseases. As therapeutic experience has shown, the meridians are inner connection tracks by which the acupuncture points are linked. Electron-microscopic examinations have shown that the acupuncture points are places with a diameter of 2–4 mm through which the molecular network of the basic regulation system penetrates through all body layers, ensuring an exchange of energy and biological information.[193]

Traditional Chinese medicine and acupuncture cannot heal cardiovascular diseases. This requires the diet and order therapy described in this book. In certain situations, however, regulations can be stabilised and complaints reduced through Chinese medicine and acupuncture.

Neural therapy

This is a highly developed art of injection therapy with local anaesthetics.
The method originates with two ingenious doctors, the brothers Ferdinand and Walter Huneke, who discovered by chance the highly regenerative effect of local anaesthesia on the affected tissue. Usually Novocain (Procain®) is injected, always without any additional substances. Novocain has three advantages as compared to local anaesthetics synthesised later in medical history: it only numbs the cellular tissue for 20 minutes, is tolerated much better by the organism, and is very quickly excreted via the kidneys into the urine without conversion by the liver. Therefore it puts no strain on the liver and metabolism. Allergic reactions have not been observed, even in persons suffering from allergies.

The substance is injected at the affected site with a very careful and highly precise injection technique. If this is done with enough time and medical sensitivity, the injections are barely painful. The method is highly efficient. With every step of the treatment, a very long-term, immediate improvement can be expected. There are three procedures with clear indications: a) purely local infiltration of the painful inflammatory tissue at the painful location, b) segment therapy, where inner organs are targeted via the reflex connections between the organs and the skin and movement segments assigned to them (via the segmental reflexes of the spinal cord) and c) interference field therapy.

The segmental therapy of the heart's sympathetic nervous system has proven very valuable for the treatment of cardiovascular diseases. The posterior roots of the sympathetic nervous system can be reached reflectorily from the vertebral joints of the 5th thoracic vertebra (points of agreement of the heart in acupuncture) and the anterior roots of the sympathetic nervous system from the reflex points at the breastbone (the alarm points of the heart and pericardium in acupuncture: points CV 17 and CV 14), which are gently injected, first superficially then more deeply. Arrhythmia can often be clearly improved by this and sometimes even eliminated. In atrial fibrillation, this therapy will reduce the pulse amplitude. This means that the degree of irregularity will decline and the patient will be much relieved. In our experience, scars from cardiac surgery, specifically of the sternum, are significant fields of interference for the heart. Their careful infiltration with Novocaine leads to a new, second more relaxed healing and always clearly improves condition and performance. An ingenious effect can often be achieved by infiltration of large ganglia (the switching stations of the vegetative nervous system that control the automatic functions).

Neural therapy cannot heal cardiovascular diseases, but it can make a valuable contribution to healing them in certain situations. Counter indications for neural therapy are strong anticoagulation with coumarines and being suffering from myasthenia.

General directives for the treatment and prevention of arteriosclerosis and cardiovascular diseases

A healing diet such as that described in this book applies a therapeutic lever to all main items at the same time: to the finest capillaries in the basic substance of the tender connective tissue and drainage of the lymphatic system, the arteries, the coronary vessels, the rennin- and aldosterone-producing kidneys, blood-pressure regulating arterioles, hormonal regulation and hormonal control of the heart by the hormones of the adrenal cortex and the thyroid, relief of the metabolism and the excretion organs, and thus regeneration of the heart muscle and readjustment of blood pressure regulation.

Seeing this diet at work in arteriosclerosis and hypertension is quite impressive. It usually reduces the increased cholesterol level within 4–7 days (regardless of the extent of the increase) and influences the increased blood pressure, except in case of pre-existing hypertension, in the sense of normalisation within 15–30 days.

This diet is very rich in fresh food. It supplies vegetable oils and fats of the highest biological quality (vegetable oils of the first cold pressing, nut butter, sesame and almond purees, whole soy, nuts, almonds, sprouted wheat, flax seed oil). The diet contains an abundance of unheated vegetables and fruit in fresh juices and salads with their blood-pressure-reducing contents. The diet uses potato salad, provides plenty of nicotinamide, vitamin B_6, and PP, vitamin E and unsaturated fatty acid, all of which reduce blood pressure. The diet virtually floods the body with citrus fruits, which are rich in vitamin C, PP and flavonoids, as well as the liver protection agent rutin, which also reduces blood pressure. The diet places high value on cultivated herbs, wild herbs, fruits, daily fresh vegetable bouillon (as a mineral-rich basis for all cooked foods), sprouted cereal grains (as an addition) and, most of all, a blood-pressure-reducing low-salt and low-sodium diet in a preparation that will bring joy to eating after a brief familiarisation period. The diet avoids almost all nutrient-rich foods and starts out with foods that are pleasantly satiating without overloading the organism with nutrients. The reduction of the usually excessive nutrient supply therefore occurs on its own. The diet greatly reduces all animal food, uses no more than 20–30 g of butter and milk fat, removes everything that is denatured and eliminates all fat from fattened animals. If the patient is not intolerant to milk protein, he may add a little animal protein in the form of buttermilk, whey, yoghurt or quark. The diet places value on tasty whole wheat cereal foods and avoids white flour and sugar.

In particular, this diet is low in table salt and can be made free of table salt or even free of sodium in patients who are particularly sensitive to salt. The diet is also particularly rich in potassium and provides the greatest possible relief for the circulation. The diet is moderate in fat and protein contents, and ensures an ideal supply thanks to an extremely economic utilisation of these two highest-quality nutrient groups. The daily fat supply, depending on the diet prescribed by the doctor, is between 10 g and 50 g, and at most 90 g. Alcohol, irritants, stimulants, tobacco, sweets and refined-flour foods must be avoided entirely. There is no diet that makes this as easy as this one does. When prepared according to the recipes in this book, the food will be tasty even without salt. The food will bring so much joy that, if necessary, such a diet may be pursued for an indeterminate period. See manual no. 9: *Enjoy food without table salt.*

The emergency regulation that becomes established during the long development period of a disease will often remain even long after the general condition has improved and the heart has recovered. It will only return to healthy regulation slowly. If the diet is interrupted in the meantime and old habits are taken up again, there may easily be new decompensations and setbacks. Therefore the patient must be aware that the relief and exercise phase of healing, which must be carefully monitored by an experienced physician, must be followed by a regeneration and stabilisation phase that requires time and consistent application. This phase often takes up to two years. Even after this, the newly learned healthy lifestyle and nutrition must be continued throughout the rest of your life. However, this is easy, once you know how good it feels to live with a healthy lifestyle.

Health of the intestines requires particular attention. The healing diet will create a physiological intestinal milieu in which the healthy intestinal flora can grow. Sometimes it must be assisted by microbial therapy to support new settlement of functional, healthy intestinal bacteria so that the putrefaction processes will end and the short-chained fatty acids and vitamin B_{12} provided by healthy intestinal flora will be produced in abundance.

A time structure that meets biological specifications and a basic reordering of lifestyle and behaviour adjusted to the natural hormonal cycles of the day/night rhythm is also very important. Heart and circulation need reliable regularity in order to regenerate. Going to bed two or (better) three hours before midnight is necessary. Breaking this rule for several nights often causes relapses. You may get up early in the morning and do the work you used to do in the evening after an early morning walk (to stimulate breathing and circulation) and a light breakfast.

There should be a break at noon, during which ideally you lie down for an hour. Two extended walks of at least one hour (total) are indispensable for healing. Longer walks or daily hiking, if possible, have an even better effect. Strenuous exercise is not sensible. Choose gradually more demanding walks in light, cool clothing.

Breathing is the only vital function that we can influence by will. Calm, deep breathing down to the abdomen may help to reduce blood pressure considerably. Practice wholly relaxed, pleasant, extended exhalation to the point where inhalation starts again involuntarily. Do these exercises several minutes every day in a relaxed position.

Where possible, practice deep relaxation. Visualize the entire weight of your body and try to perceive its complete heaviness. Imagine taking this weight down onto your bed or couch until, as a sign of relaxation, pleasant warmth spreads in the limbs. Practice this many times until it is easy.

Equally important, morning skin care should include dry brushing and rubbing the skin with a moist wash cloth.

You can also perform your own hydrotherapy. In the case of a heavy, full abdomen, a nightly body compress will provide simple and effective help. In a body compress, the blood pressure drops sharply at night, and a pleasant relaxation ensues. Arm baths with increasing temperature relieve blood pressure and the heart simply and effectively: place your arms in a bath of 36 °C up to the middle of the upper arm and increase the temperature slowly by adding hot water (42° to 45 °C) for at least 7 minutes until you start to sweat slightly. After another 10 minutes, rest lightly covered. Do the same with your feet to the middle of the calves, or at the same time with the arms and feet.

Sun baths are very valuable for healing, except in cases of hypertension, if starting with 5 minutes each side of the body and gradually increasing to 15 minutes per side. The head should be covered and no sunscreen should be used, since the effect of the UV-B spectrum of sunlight would be filtered out. After every sunbath, you should wash with cool water and rest.

It is also very important to protect yourself from mental stress. As far as possible, try to stay away from situations with a tense atmosphere, avoid stressful discussions, and stay away from situations that create tension and anger. Avoid social idleness, especially by going to bed late, and endeavour to spend an hour alone every day, during which you can order and evaluate your thoughts and feelings. Consciously guide your attention towards constructive and joyful thinking.

The healing regime

As we have seen, cardiovascular diseases are created on the basis of a general disorder of lifestyle and nutrition. If you want to prevent arteriosclerosis with all of its dangerous complications such as heart attack and stroke, and if you want to remove the changes in the arterial walls that start in early childhood, you will have to let go of current ideas and presumed social obligations and take your own life in hand and reorder it, just as it corresponds to our biological nature. Thus the organism is given back the prerequisites it needs to remove the disorder in the metabolism that has resulted from them and the dangerous slagging of the matrix of the intercellular tissue, and to recover the highly complex and ingenuously designed regulatory capacity of our biological system.

No social event or party today still demands that alcohol be drunk and unhealthy snacks be eaten. Quite the opposite: the old celebration of togetherness with the drinking of wine, beer and spirits has become a banality and a silent, elegant abstinence has come to be seen as refined restraint that often brings secret admiration. It may happen that some events become boring, since the stupid, overly loud talk of those who are drinking alcohol will neither raise interest nor bring joy. Your own thoughts will remain clear and cannot be deceived.

During work breaks it may help to remember that coffee will only briefly reduce the mental inertia and irritability that it has produced in the long term, to then leave behind even more exhaustion, irritability and mental inertia. It also helps to remember that coffee and alcohol strongly facilitate certain kinds of cancer.

Many things stimulate appetite, especially food that is roasted or baked in fat, as well as industrial food products to which appetising substances have been added. Chocolate, sweets, salty or cheese pastry also artificially stimulate the appetite. If you have previously been trapped into the poor nutrition that is so popular today, your own sense of taste, dulled and atrophied, will be accustomed to these excessive flavours.

Your feeling of satiation will also be atrophied, and often you will only feel sated when your stomach and metabolism have been filled and overloaded with senselessly supplied nutrients. Often attacks of ravenous hunger come about, with snacking to fill up the inner void, which in turn increases these ravenous attacks in a kind of vicious circle. Then the natural regulation mechanisms for appetite and body weight break down, and most suffer from grotesque obesity, while other individuals emaciate and wither, depending on their constitution.

The body must learn to remove all of these deeply rooted impairments. You must learn a new appetite behaviour, not only by eating with the palate and sense of smell, but also by choosing the quantity and composition of your food with the sensations of your entire body. In the stomach, in the intestine, in all cell tissues, down to the fingers and the tips of your toes, you can feel if a food has stressed you or been well tolerated. This is a new, original second type of appetite and satiation behaviour that has previously been lost through years of biologically poor nutrition. Inner warming and blood pressure increased from a meal rich in protein and salt were usually misinterpreted as increased energy. The fatigue caused by such meals were misunderstood as satiety and covered over with a cup of coffee.

All of these misinterpretations and the impaired appetite behaviour can best be removed by making use of holiday time to start your new, ordered lifestyle. If you used to smoke, you should reduce your consumption by one cigarette a day until you reach five a day and eliminate alcohol altogether. Getting rid of smoking and alcohol entirely is a natural prerequisite for the prevention and healing of cardiovascular diseases. Particularly with smoking, but also with alcohol, there will be an enormous chemical dependency that often requires in-patient treatment for withdrawal. During this treatment, dietetic therapy may be started.

The practical application of the healing diet

After a careful review of the metabolism, we usually start with the first diet stage. If there is any diabetes, gout or kidney damage, the metabolism change must be slower, i.e. with the second-stage diet, under careful monitoring of the lab values by the attending physician. For this, we refer to our detailed instructions in the Bircher-Benner manual no. 4 here: *Fresh juices, raw vegetables and fruit dishes*, which we urgently recommend for careful study.

Some people have made the experience that they tolerated raw food badly. If the intestinal milieu is alkaline because of high protein consumption, there will always be a more or less poor bacterial settlement in the large intestine, and often the small intestine and the stomach too, with anaerobic germs that produce putrefaction gases and often permit fungal infection. These persons usually suffer from flatulence, heart burn and irregular stool. This kind of impaired intestinal milieu is a huge field of interference and is not prepared for digesting raw food, which at first may increase flatulence and feeling. unwell This rather common situation may reliably be overcome after two or three weeks of the first-stage diet with our fresh juice and almond milk. Afterwards the raw food will be tolerated easily. Note the Bircher-Benner manual no. 14: *Manual for patients with gastrointestinal conditions*.

Our diet stages I to III are a vegan healing diet that leads to pervasive regeneration and detoxing of all tissues. Stage IV is a full regime rich in raw food with a careful addition of up to 30 g of fresh butter or cream, buttermilk, yoghurt or quark. It is used for further healing and maintaining health after an individual duration of the prior vegan diet stages I to III.

For the metabolism, the vegan raw food of stages I and II is extremely economic, since it supplies all the important nutritional, vital substances and minerals that we need in perfect composition and bioavailability, without any stressful excess. These diet levels provide the highest energy potential for regeneration. They protect and regenerate the digestive organs and particularly the liver and kidneys that are so important for lipid metabolism and blood-pressure regulation. Additionally, this diet causes rapid, extremely intense diuresis (excretion of water and toxins) from all tissues and thus quick relief for the heart and circulation.

The intestinal flora is slowly regenerated so that the putrefaction-producing anaerobic bacteria and candida fungi inside the intestine are replaced by aerobic ones and displace other pathogenic germs. Pathological Escherichia coli strains are replaced by healthy ones. This is reflected by the stool turning soft and yellowish. The dietary fibre of vegetable food will be degraded into short-chained fatty acids by the healthy intestinal flora, particularly butyric acid, which is very important for feeding the cells of the intestinal mucosa and protects it from developing cancer.

Inflammation in the intestine is reduced and the mucosa is covered by a protective mucous layer with a high content of IgA antibodies that enable the lymphocytes of the enteral immune systems to differentiate clearly between what is alien and what is not again. In this way the immune system will be supplied with optimally immunocompetent cells only after just a few weeks, so that allergies and autoimmune reactions will slowly be reduced over the course of several months.

Raw food enables the basic system of the soft connective tissue to excrete the deposited metabolic wastes such as degenerative proteins, amyloids and oxidised lipids and such as oxidised LDL cholesterol through the lymphatic pathways. This will restore the function of the proteoglycan network as a molecular screen and a storage and conductive system for biological information from month to month. The regulatory ability will therefore slowly return.

The red blood corpuscles will be able to deform when passing the capillaries again after only a few days of raw food diet. This will provide a high-quality oxygen supply to all body tissues so that they can regenerate. The blood will be less viscose and the danger of thrombosis and embolism will decline.

If there are any food intolerances, after comprehensive allergy testing we will develop an individual dietary plan that is to be complied with until the intolerances have disappeared.

If dangerous arteriosclerosis foci are already present, the raw food diet of stages I and II must be maintained for many months so that they will decline as quickly as possible. If the hypertension is not yet persistent, normal values will appear in sleep and when relaxed. In this case, hypertension will usually decrease within a few weeks. The raw food regime should be continued until the blood pressure has been completely normalised. Blood pressure reducing agents can be reduced slowly and finally discontinued in this situation, under the supervision of the attending physician. For persistent hypertension with consistently high values, healing will take many months, often up to two years, since the structural changes will have to reverse first. Much will be gained if the diet stages I and II are continued as long as possible. Then you can move on to the third diet stage, although you may insert raw food weeks every once in a while. The proportion of cooked food should never exceed one third of a meal.

The fourth low salt diet stage with a little buttermilk, sour milk, yoghurt and no more than 30 g of fresh butter or cream will also contribute to the healing of the arteries. It is very pleasant to the taste and therefore very suitable as a permanent regime. It should only be started when the blood pressure has normalised and no considerable constrictions are evident in the arteries anymore.

The diet stages
Stage I diet
The fresh juice and almond milk regime
The fruit cells are broken down in the juices freshly prepared with the centrifugal juicer. They are very rich in vitamins, enzymes and secondary plant substances with their inherent pharmacological effects. The plant fibres of the cell walls are partially removed. In this form, vegetarian raw food is very easy to digest and will lead to the fastest change of the milieu in the gastrointestinal tract and the metabolism. Prepared fresh and correctly, almond milk is very pleasant to drink. It is similar to breast milk in composition and contains essential, polyunsaturated fatty acids that complement the powerful antioxidative effect of the fresh fruit juices. Additionally, at least twice a day 2 tablespoons of fresh, cold-pressed flax seed oil should either be mixed into the juices or at stage II in the Birchermuesli and the salad dressing or consumed directly from a spoon. This is very important to ensure a satisfactory supply of omega-3 fatty acids and a correct ratio of omega-6/omega-3 fatty acids. The juices must always be fresh, drunk right from the centrifugal juicer, in order to have their full energy potential. They should be enjoyed slowly, sip by sip. If you do not tolerate the fruit acid well at first, add one third rice gruel. You can also mix in a little banana to bind the fruit acid. If weight reduction is not required, you may also eat unroasted almonds, nuts, sunflower seeds, pine nuts and pumpkin seeds. Manual no. 4 describes this regime in detail. We recommend that you read it. The diet is as follows:

Morning and evening

2 different fruit juices freshly prepared with the centrifugal juicer
1 almond milk
almonds and nuts
herbal tea

Lunch

2 different fruit juices
1 vegetable juice
almonds and nuts
herbal tea

Usually two dl per juice are sufficient to quell hunger. Otherwise the volume may be increased. You may also replace one or both fruit juices with vegetable juice or mix various fruits and vegetables. The earthy taste of the root vegetables can be made more palatable with the addition of sun-ripened fruit (e.g. beetroot juice with a little pineapple or pear, carrot juice with apple). You may also be creative in your mixes. A very popular mix is carrot with celery, tomato and a pinch of raw potato or fennel. Salad leaves such as spinach, head lettuce, endives, etc. are valuable and may contribute to interesting and delicious juice mixtures, as would the addition of a little onion or a very little garlic, both particularly valuable for healing arteriosclerosis. Between meals you may drink all kinds of teas, but they should not be black or green teas because of the caffeine content. If your stomach is irritated, a small raw potato can be added with an apple. Drunk slowly, this will reduce heart

burn. Always add one third rice or barley gruel to all juices until your stomach has become calmer. We recommend manual no. 14: *Manual for patients with gastrointestinal conditions*. It contains valuable explanations and tables of suitable vegetables and fruits that soothe the stomach (for digestive problems too). Suitable fresh herbs may be placed in the vegetable juice for decoration. If you wish you may also follow up the juice meal with a vegetable bouillon with fresh herbs, made from fresh vegetables, once or twice a day, as long as it is cooked without salt.
Raw potatoes must be used only in small amounts (1 small potato per meal), because of the solanine content.

Low blood sugar may manifest itself, especially around day three, causing you to feel unwell and weak. Therefore we recommend that you have a few raisins on hand at all times. Raisins may be eaten at any time and will quickly eliminate the problem. Such changes in the metabolism often become evident around the third day. If you are working, you should switch to stage II for 1–3 days from day three onwards, to make these reactions less of a problem. Manual no. 4 provides valuable information on these matters. If you were still drinking coffee when you started the diet, you may have a headache as a withdrawal symptom. This will disappear after 2 or 3 days. During this diet stage you should rest a lot, alternating rest with brief walks. We recommend assistance by a doctor familiar with this therapy.

Stage II diet
The vegetable fresh food diet

This stage naturally continues the healing of the intestinal milieu and metabolism already initiated and assures a full capacity for work. You may be a bit dreamier during the raw food regime, but your mental and physical powers will nevertheless be more than adequate. You will find access to suppressed emotions and dreams more easily, so that you can process them with renewed and improved acuity. Apart from this, your mood will be brightened. The important rule of bedtime before midnight must be complied with under all circumstances. During sleep after midnight, dream experiences will deepen and the dreams will be more accessible to your consciousness. This serves to keep your soul healthy but helps rather less with your recuperation.

Breakfast and dinner

Birchermuesli with 2 tablespoons of flax seed oil, which can also be taken separately
almond milk
almonds and nuts
herbal tea

Lunch

Begin lunch with fruit (e.g. fruit or vegetable juice), then have some almond milk, nuts and almonds, with tea or water.

Next have a gaily garnished raw food dish with a salad of a root vegetable, a second dish of leaf salad and a third one of a vegetable fruit (e.g. tomato, cucumber), to combine all nutritious contents. Create a decorative colour combination, and enrich the raw food dish with fresh herbs and matching nuts or seeds. If tolerated, add fresh onions and a little fresh garlic. If you like, you may then have a salt free bouillon made of fresh vegetables and garnished with fresh herbs.

The recipe part contains tried and tested weekly regimes and interesting recipes, including recipes for salad dressings, which must be prepared according to these instructions.

Stage III diet

After staying with the raw food diet for sufficiently long, you may switch to this vegan diet level when you desire hot food. The vegan diet corresponds to the level–II diet but includes gently steamed vegetables with a small portion of potatoes in their jackets or mashed potatoes or whole rice, buckwheat, quinoa or maize after the raw food for lunch. The share of hot foods should be eaten after the raw food and not exceed one-third of the entire lunch. The vegetable portion should prevail. You should note that your weight will no longer decline at this diet stage. You need to return repeatedly to pure raw food for many days or weeks, until your ideal weight is reached if you are suffering from obesity. On raw food days, you may still fulfil your desire for hot food with the vegetable bouillon and hot tea. During this and the next diet stage, it is very important for regulation of the gastrointestinal tract and metabolism to remember to keep the meals small and to take them slowly and to chew them carefully. If you no longer need to lose weight, you may have a little wholemeal bread with nut butter for breakfast and dinner.

Stage IV diet
This is a modern vegetarian full dietary regime that continues to satisfy the latest insights from nutritional science. It corresponds to the Stage III diet, but permits up to 30 g of fresh butter or fresh cream, buttermilk, natural yoghurt and quark. Nut butter is preferred to fresh butter. This diet stage is no healthier than level III. However, it permits more diversity and thus is very pleasant and appetising, while still suitable for preventing cardiovascular diseases and maintaining general health.

However, industrial processing of cow's milk, and particularly homogenisation and ultra-high-temperature processing, have caused a great many people to become intolerant to milk today. Butter, whole cream and condensed milk are tolerated better than homogenised, pasteurised milk, yoghurt and quark. Intolerances are often misinterpreted as lactose intolerance. For homogenisation, the fresh milk is pressurised at 5 atmospheres and then sprayed onto a hot plate. This changes the spatial structure of the large molecules so that the milk fat can no longer turn to cream. The immune cells of the enteral immune systems will recognise such crippled protein molecules as suspicious and report them to the antibody-producing B-cells, which will form immune antibodies of type IgG4, the cause of more-or-less strong milk intolerance. You may feel a paradoxical yearning for milk, or a revulsion to milk, or simply unspecific digestive problems after eating milk, buttermilk, quark or yoghurt, up to stomach ache or slight diarrhoea. The IgE antibodies against albumin and milk globulins are usually not yet apparent. They would be signs of a massive allergy to milk protein.

Milk intolerance can usually be recorded by anamnesis. If there is any doubt, allergy testing is required. If it is present, it will be worthwhile to stay with the third, vegan diet stage, which will make you feel much better and will better advance healing.

If you continue a vegan diet for a long time, the vitamin B_{12} level must be monitored. In healthy intestinal flora, bacteria in the large intestine will produce vitamin B_{12}. Nevertheless, a long-term vegan diet will usually keep the vitamin B_{12} level slightly below the official standard of people who also eat dairy products and meat, but without producing any sign of B_{12} deficit in the blood count or even in the form of the dangerous sensitivity disorder of the feet. Instead of vitamin tablets, vitamin B_{12} can be supplied by biological yeast extract or hawthorn, which is a very valuable plant that contains vegetable vitamin B_{12}.

Secondary plant substances

Vegetable food contains substances with pharmacological effects. These are called secondary plant substances, or phytochemicals. Animal food contains no substances with pharmacological effect. Bircher-Benner manual no. 4 describes them in detail.

In the diet to prevent and heal arteriosclerosis, hypertension and cardiovascular diseases, it is worthwhile favouring foods that are particularly rich in suitable secondary plant substances.

Foods with a particularly strong antioxidative effect

All fruits and vegetables are rich in flavonoids and carotenoids (xanthines) with strong antioxidative effects. Flavonoids are present in the outer layers of vegetables and fruit and will be lost when peeling. The effect of carotenoids is lost when cooking.

On raw food therapy to prevent thrombosis and embolism

Raw onions and garlic prevent blood clots, as do flavonoid-containing vegetables and fruits because of their high polyphenol content. These foods inhibit the aggregation of blood platelets (thrombocyte aggregation inhibition).[194] In garlic containing ajoene, this effect is strongest and comparable to the effective strength of aspirin (acetyl salicylic acid).[195]

Ajoen can only be found in fresh garlic. Garlic powder and extracts, sautéed and roasted garlic are ineffective in this respect. Ajoen of garlic and allicin of fresh onion inhibit thrombocyte aggregation via inhibition of enzymes for the formation of thromboxane (catalysing) just like the flavonoids of fruits and vegetables and the sulphides of onion plants. Similar effects on blood platelet aggregation have been documented as well for the polyphenols of the outer layers of fruits and vegetables. In an epidemiological study, patients with cardiovascular disease who had the highest flavonoid intake through citrus and fruits in their nutrition showed the lowest mortality rate.[192] Flavonoids are lost entirely by peeling fruit and partially through storage, but they survive cooking.

Special Features of Raw Food Therapy for Hypertension

Fibre-rich (plant) nutrition lowers blood pressure by various mechanisms.[196] Some dietary fibre is broken down by intestinal bacteria into short-chained fatty acids that lower blood pressure. Pectins are water-soluble dietary fibres in apples, bananas and citrus fruits with blood pressure reducing effects. Caffeine and theophylline from coffee and black tea displace adenosine from its receptors at the cells and thus increase blood pressure. At the brain neurons, adenosine will block the entrance of information into the brain cells (neurons) when there is overload of the nervous system to protect them from exhaustion. Caffeine blocks the adenosine receptors. Drinking coffee continually sabotages this important protective mechanism of the brain cells and thus causes them to become dangerously exhausted in the long run. Blood pressure reducing substances were extracted from garlic, including adenosine and allicin. This effect of fresh garlic can help to treat hypertension.

Special Features of Raw Food Therapy for the Reduction of Cholesterol Levels

Cholesterol is formed in the liver and serves as a basic substance for the synthesis of the primary bile acids and steroid hormones (cortisol, sex hormones). Vegetable foods do not contain cholesterol but do have cholesterol-reducing ingredients. The saponins of the legumes reduce cholesterol by reducing its resorption in the intestine. The primary bile acids are synthesised from cholesterol by the liver and emitted through the biliary ducts into the intestine for fat resorption, after which they return to the liver through the portal vein as fat mycelia (enterohepatic cycle). Only a small part of the primary bile acids is converted into secondary bile acids by the bacterial flora in the intestine and then excreted. The saponins increase this extrusion by saponification and thus effectively reduce cholesterol. Beans and lucerne are particularly rich in saponins. Cold-pressed vegetable oils contain phytosterins. They reduce cholesterol levels in various ways.[197]

Tocotrienols of the whole grain seeds of rye, barley and oats, palm oil, oat oil and barley oil inhibit the synthesis of cholesterol. Allicin from garlic, the carotenoids of fruits and vegetables, vitamins C and E and anthocyanins of aubergines reduce LDL cholesterol (low density cholesterol) effectively without influencing HDL cholesterol. We have seen that LDL cholesterol does not cause arteriosclerosis unless oxidised (made rancid) on the way from the liver to the cell tissues by the oxidative stress of poor nutrition and lifestyle, and that it is extremely important for the memory and membrane stability of all cellular tissues. In contrast to statin medication, the vegetable diet will not reduce the LDL cholesterol too far, but to an ideal degree, protecting it reliably from dangerous oxidation at the same time with its strong antioxidant effect.

Very often, cardiovascular diseases coincide with type 2 diabetes. The vegetable raw food regime protects from diabetes very effectively. See our Bircher-Benner manuals no. 4 and no. 7. At the same time, the vegetable raw food regime offers excellent protection from obesity as a risk factor for cardiovascular diseases, and from anorexia. See our Bircher-Benner manuals no. 14 and 26.

The recipe section contains tried and tested and well-tolerated recipes from the world-renowned Bircher-Benner Centre for Scientific Natural Medicine as well as weekly regimes to make the diet easier to follow.

Menu

Menus for various rawfood regimes

1. Fresh Juice Fasting (bed/juice day)

Morning and evening
    200 g fruit juice

Lunch
    200 g fruit juice or
    200 g seasonal vegetable juice (tomato or carrot juice, or a mix of tomato, carrot and spinach juice)
    Orange and tangerine juice
    grapefruit juice
    berry juices
    grape juice
    plum juice
    peach juice
    apricot juice
    Japanese persimmon juice
    fresh apple and pear juice

These juices can also be combined (e.g. berry with peach or apricot juice, apricot with orange juice, apple with pear juice).

Many people suffer from gastritis or stomach ulcers, often without knowing it. They are usually sensitive to fruit acids and therefore should avoid raw fruit. Such patients, however, need completely fresh fruit; citric acid, racemic acid and malic acid are particularly valuable for them. If the fruit acids are bound suitably by adding cereal gruel, they will be easily tolerated (see recipe for gruels).

Depending on doctor's orders, fresh juice fasting may be undertaken for one or several days – even two, three or (rarely) four weeks. Medical supervision during fasting and subsequent recuperation is important (see table on page 130). If only mild effects of fasting are desired – in the sense of general detoxification, dewatering and rejuvenation – a strict fruit juice day can be used once a week within the raw food treatment or regular diet where complete rest (preferably bed rest) is possible. If you do not rest during the first one or two fasting days, the full effect will be impaired by fatigue and hunger, and there will not be proper relaxation and urine flow. Do not be deterred by reactions such as headache, nausea, pain in the limbs, and weakness (especially in the afternoon). These show that the body is doing its detoxification work during juice fasting, so that such days have meaning and purpose. However, be sure to report your observations to your doctor.

2. Full Juice Day

High quality, relatively nutritious food is administered. This regime can be maintained for one week or longer with the addition of cereal gruels, and can be prolonged for several weeks with the avoidance of extreme physical and mental stress. Full juice periods are suitable to start readjustment treatment, for dewatering and weight loss treatments, or if the organism is very low in respect of vital substance (e.g. in the case of chronic digestive diseases), as a sequel to a traditional bland raw food free diet. In such cases, fruit juice should initially be taken with ⅓ flax seed, barley or rice gruel. For dewatering treatments, urine and weight must be measured at regular intervals. If necessary, water-expelling tea (solidago, rosehip) must be drunk.

Morning

200 to 400 g	fruit juice (two different juices)
150 to 200 g	almond milk
1 cup	rosehip tea

Lunch

200 to 400 g	fruit juice (two different juices)
200 g	vegetable juice
150–200 g	almond milk

Evening
Same as in the morning

3. Fruit Fasting Days

Fruit fasting may replace juice fasting in bed (the strict form of the fruit juice fasting day), e.g. when metabolism change and stimulation of the intestine by cellulose content is the principal aim, rather than protection through free cellulose. Since this diet produces a strong feeling of satiation, fruit fasting can be performed even on days without complete rest, and for extended periods of time. The effect of juice fasting is, however, more intense. Fruit fasting is indicated for persons with heart disease, chronic liver weakness, or lazy bowels. Other indications are an apple day for acute diarrhea and a strawberry day for celiac disease and abdominal congestion. Duration: 1–5 days (longer if prescribed by the doctor). We refer here to the Bircher-Benner manual no. 14: Manual for patients with gastrointestinal conditions.

Daily menu: 3 times 200–250 g (up to 300 g) washed, fresh, completely ripe, unsweetened fruit, e.g. berries, citrus fruit (oranges, grapefruit, tangerines), grapes, figs, melons, Japanese persimmons.

Special fruit fasting forms
Apple day
1–6 times 1 large apple finely ground for acute gastrointestinal catarrh with diarrhoea.

Strawberry day
3–4 times 200–250 g very ripe strawberries, unsweetened, for celiac disease (special form of chronic diarrhoea) and vitamin-C deficit.

Blueberry day
3 times 200–250 g for slight intestinal infection. Slightly congestive.

Blackberry day
3 times 200–250 g completely ripe blackberries. Particularly rich in natural sugar and vitamin C. Nutritious and easy to digest.

Currant day
3 times 200–250 g ($2/3$ red and yellow, $1/3$ black). For patients with liver problems. Particularly refreshing and thirst relieving. Rich in vitamin C.

Japanese persimmon day
2 small (or 1 large) Japanese persimmon fruits, 4 times a day. Very nutritious and rich in vitamins C and B.

Grape day (traditional grape treatment)
750–1000 g sun-ripened grapes, if possible untreated, distributed over 4–5 meals per day. Wash thoroughly and clean of treatment residue (briefly flush in hot water). Eat whole fruit. Low in vitamins, but particularly nutritious because of its high fruit sugar content. Liver protection! Stimulates intestine with seeds. Duration: 1–2 weeks, longer if prescribed by doctor (up to 6 weeks).

Fig day
3 times 200 g fresh figs. Stimulates the intestine. Nutritious. No more than 1 day.

4. Raw Vegetable Menus (for stage II diet)

Below are seven examples of raw vegetable combinations for lunch for each season. (Special value is placed on the harmonious distribution of bulb, root and leaf raw vegetables, but always use them fresh and quite ripe.) For a full daily menu, see page 98.

a) *Spring*
1st day: fruits – nuts (also dried fruit) – radishes – fennel – head lettuce
2nd day: fruits – nuts – celery roots (celeriac) – tomatoes – cress
3rd day: fruit – nuts – carrots – chicory/endive – head lettuce
4th day: fruit – nuts – radish – lettuce – cress
5th day: fruits – nuts – beetroot – dandelion – head lettuce
6th day: fruits – nuts – cauliflower – spinach – cress
7th day: fruits – nuts – kohlrabi – tomatoes – head lettuce

b) *Summer*
1st day: fruits – nuts – radish – tomatoes – head lettuce
2nd day: fruits – nuts – carrots – courgettes – head lettuce
3rd day: fruits – nuts – cauliflower – radishes – head lettuce
4th day: fruits – nuts – kohlrabi – cress – head lettuce
5th day: fruits – nuts – celery – lettuce – head lettuce
6th day: fruits – nuts – tomatoes stuffed with cauliflower – head lettuce
7th day: fruits – nuts – small beets – cucumbers – head lettuce

c) *Autumn*
1st day: fruits – nuts – celery – tomatoes – endives
2nd day: fruits – nuts – beetroot – peppers – head lettuce
3rd day: fruits – nuts – black salsify – spinach – head lettuce
4th day: fruits – nuts – cauliflower – lamb's lettuce – endives
5th day: fruits – nuts – small beets – courgettes – cress
6th day: fruits – nuts – radish – tomatoes – head lettuce
7th day: fruits – nuts – celery (celeriac) – cucumber – head lettuce

d) *Winter*
1st day: fruits – nuts – black salsify – red cabbage – endives
2nd day: fruits – nuts – celery – radicchio – head lettuce
3rd day: fruits – nuts – carrots – peppers – head lettuce
4th day: fruits – nuts – beetroot – sauerkraut – endives
5th day: fruits – nuts – cauliflower – spinach – lamb's lettuce
6th day: fruits – nuts – tomatoes – chicory – head lettuce

Daily menu

Breakfast

Birchermuesli	120–200 g
Ground almonds or hazelnuts	20–30 g
Fruits	100–200 g
Optional rosehip tea	1 cup

If a mushy or liquid consistency is desired:
Birchermuesli with finely ground or mixed fruits and with almond milk (20–30 g almond puree)
150 g fruit juice
1 cup of rosehip tea

The quantities need only approximate to those indicated. What is important is the natural feeling that must not be impaired by stimulants or habits. Only where very litttle nutrition is desired should hunger be reduced by long chewing and salivation and by a slower intake of food. In some cases, a little fresh cream that has not been subjected to UHT-processing can be added, where noted below. This is particularly sensible when underweight. It may also be replaced by almond puree.

Lunch

Fruits or chilled fruit soup	150–250 g
Green lettuce	50–100 g
Raw vegetable plate	approx. 100–150 g
Nuts of all kinds	approx. 20 g
1 glass of unfermented apple or grape juice (optional)	200 g

or

Fruit juice	approx. 100–200 g
Green lettuce, finely chopped	approx. 50 g
Raw vegetables blended or mashed (cucumbers, tomatoes)	100 g
Vegetable juice (spinach, carrots, etc.) with a touch of cream or almond puree and lemon juice	100 g
Almond milk or sesame milk	approx. 200 g
Optional apple or grape juice	200 g

Evening meal

Birchermuesli	150–200 g
Nuts	20–30 g
Fruits	100–20 g
Optional rosehip tea	1 cup

or

Birchermuesli	150–200 g
Almond milk	approx. 200 g
Fruit juice	approx. 200 g
Optional rosehip tea	1 cup

5. Raw Food Day with Side Dish

Morning and evening
Same as raw food day

Lunch
Fruits, nuts
Raw vegetable plate
2 dl vegetable bouillon
2 baked potatoes (see recipe page 120)

6. Transitional Food

Breakfast
Birchermuesli with ground nuts
2 slices of wholemeal bread or crispbread
Approx. 15 g butter
Fruits
Herbal tea, or milk or yoghurt

Lunch
Fruits
Raw vegetables: cauliflower, spinach, head lettuce
Potato soup
Steamed tomato, vegetables
Whole rice, only with fresh butter or a little olive oil, no cheese, lightly salted

Dinner
Same as breakfast
Optional rosehip jam or honey as bread spread

The Recipes

A healing regime for patients with high blood pressure or arteriosclerosis requires strict attention to the use of salt. Diet stages I and II do not allow any salt at all. Afterwards, and in the later everyday regime, salt should be used very sparingly. Normal table salt is unsuitable. Sea salt would be better, but because of the general pollution of the sea (i.e. chemicals and radioactive substances) sea salt cannot be recommended. The best alternative is Tibetan or European rock salt. Spices like yeast extracts, soy sauce and Kelpamare must be used with care as well. They contain relatively large amounts of salt. There are only very few salt-free ones (e.g. Herbamare and Plantaforce by Vogel). Caution: yeast extract is allowed as a cover name for harmful glutamate. It is best to ask for advice in a health-food store. Japanese miso (fermented soybean paste) is a salt free spice. However, since the nuclear disaster of Fukushima, Japanese products must be used cautiously. Today a lot of soy is produced by genetic modification. Products free of genetically modified organisms are marked with the organic bud.

Our recipes need only very little rock salt or spice. The salads use no salt at all. Thanks to the imaginative use of herbs and other spices (onions, garlic, celery leaves, etc.), the dishes are delicious.

Juices are from raw fruits and vegetables in a mechanically refined form, used as additional special enrichment and for patients with gastrointestinal diseases, when coarse food (cellulose) is not permitted. Whole raw vegetables are always higher in nutritional quality and cannot be permanently replaced by juice.

For the preparation of juices, raw vegetables must be cleaned thoroughly, pressed with a hand press or an electrical centrifugal juicer, and served immediately. Any resting time reduces their value.

Fruit Juices

Unmixed fruit juices
Orange, tangerine, grapefruit, apple, pear, grape, strawberry, blueberry, currant, cassis, raspberry, peach, apricot, plum, mango, Japanese persimmon, kiwi.

Mixed fruit juices
Orange, tangerine, grapefruit, Japanese persimmon or berry juice with apple juice (or berry juice with peach), apricot or plum juice (or mashed bananas) with orange, berry, peach, mango or apricot juice.

Optional: lemon juice, honey, maple syrup, fruit concentrate, yoghurt, almond milk. If underweight and if milk protein is tolerated, you may add a little cream.

Vegetable Juices

When fresh they have a high mineral and vitamin content. Each juice has its own special value.

Unmixed vegetable juices
Tomato, carrot, beetroot, radish, cabbage, celery, and all leaf, bulb and root vegeta-

bles; stinging nettle, sorrel and dandelion juice for springtime blood-cleansing treatment.

Mixed vegetable juices
Carrot, tomato, and spinach in equal proportions (very delicious)
tomato and carrot
tomato and spinach.

Other mixes (and cocktails) can be combined according to taste.

For variety, add sorrel, stinging nettle, chives, parsley, onions, tender celery leaves or roots, and other herbs.

Additions per glass (1½–2 dl): 1 teaspoon almond puree or if tolerated, 1 tablespoon buttermilk, lemon juice, or some fruit concentrate (optional).

Potato Juice

Prepare scrubbed, peeled (optional) small potatoes (no unripe, green or sprouted ones) like carrot juice. Not tasty, but relieves cramps and is particularly effective for heartburn and for stomach and duodenal ulcers. The flavour can be improved by adding an apple to the juicer.

Gruel to Accompany Juices

The gruel is added to raw juices in a proportion of 1:3. It neutralises the sharpness of the fruit or vegetable flavour. The daily ration can be prepared once a day and kept in a thermos bottle.

Rice or barley gruel:
Stir 1 heaped teaspoon rice or barley wholemeal flour with 2 dl cold water and boil for 5 min., stirring constantly. Let cool.

Flax seed gruel:
Rinse 1 tablespoon flax seed, boil in 2 dl water for 10 min., strain and let cool.

Birchermuesli

All recipes are for 1 person.

Birchermuesli
In our long experience, the original apple muesli as invented by Dr. Bircher and used successfully thousands of times with his patients has remained the best food for the regime. This used to be called fruit dish (Früchtespeise). Called d'Spys by the patients, it soon conquered the world under the name of Birchermuesli.

Sweet-sour juicy apples with white flesh are best for the muesli (e.g. Klar, Gravenstein, Sauergrauech, Menznauer Jäger, Jonathan, Ontario, Rubinette, Glockenäpfel, Braeburn, Champagner-Reinetten, Cox's Orange).

The flavour of drier apple types with a weaker taste can be enriched with a pinch of freshly ground peel of untreated orange or lemon, or with orange juice, a little rosehip paste or freshly ground ginger.

Birchermuesli with almond or sesame puree
1 tablespoon oat flakes
3 tablespoons water
½ tablespoon lemon juice
1 tablespoon almond or sesame puree
1 tablespoon honey
3 tablespoons water
200 g apples
1 tablespoon hazelnuts or almonds, ground

Soak oat flakes or freshly chopped oats for 12 hours so that the resulting oat gruel will absorb the fruit acids. Rapid flakes do not need to soak for as long. Stir in lemon

juice, puree, honey and water with a whisk to produce a creamy consistency, add the oat flakes and grate apples with the Bircher grater. Stir in at once. Spread nuts on top, decorate with fruit cut to size or berries and nuts. Serve at once.
Versions: Replace oat flakes with wheat, rice, barley, rye, semolina, buckwheat or soy flakes, optionally mixed with yeast flakes (enriching with vitamin B_{12}).

Another version: Mix 1 teaspoon soaked oat flakes with 1 teaspoon cereal grains (whole, chopped or mixed). Soak in water for 24 hrs. then put through a sieve and rinse with cold water.

Birchermuesli with yoghurt, sour milk or buttermilk
1 tablespoon oat flakes
3 tablespoon water
2 tablespoon Bifidus yoghurt, Bifidus sour milk or buttermilk
1 teaspoon honey
200 g apples
1 tablespoon hazelnuts or almonds, ground

Soak the oat flakes for 12 hours (overnight if for breakfast). Mix the oat flakes, yoghurt (or sour milk) and honey into a smooth sauce. Remove stems and calyxes from the washed apples and grate the apples with the Bircher grater into the sauce. Stir several times to keep the muesli pleasantly white. Spread the nuts on it and serve at once. Never let it rest.

Birchermuesli with orange juice
1 tablespoon (8 g) fine oat flakes
3 tablespoons water
$1/2$ tablespoon lemon juice
$1/2$ orange, squeezed
200 g apples
1 tablespoon hazelnuts or almonds, ground

Prepared like basic recipe.

Birchermuesli with berries or stone fruit
(particularly rich in vitamin C)

Prepare an almond-puree, sesame-puree or yoghurt sauce. Add 150–200 g strawberries or raspberries, blueberries, currants or blackberries, and mash slightly with a fork.
Or
150–200 g plums, peaches or apricots, pitted and passed through the chopper or cut finely with a knife. Avoid plums and apricots for patients with chronic diarrhoea. We refer here to the Bircher-Benner manual no. 14: Manual for patients with gastrointestinal conditions.

Birchermuesli with various fruits
The following combinations are very tasty:

strawberries and raspberries
strawberries, raspberries and currants
strawberries and apples
blackberries and apples
apples with finely cut orange and tangerine segments
apples and bananas
apples and peaches
sauce: almond or sesam puree sauce, or yoghurt sauce
Use only fresh fruits, never use canned fruits (fruit salad, etc.).

Birchermuesli with dried fruits
If you have no fresh fruits on hand, you can also make the muesli with dried fruits (apples, apricots, plums, pears). One hundred grams of dried fruits are washed, soaked in cold water for 12 hours and passed through the chopper. Mix with almond or sesame puree sauce or yoghurt sauce. For dried fruits, always look for good quality without preservatives or bleach; otherwise, gastrointestinal problems may occur. Dried fruits do not have the full energy potential of fresh fruit.

Birchermuesli with condensed milk

If you do not have almond or sesame puree or fresh yoghurt to hand, you can make the muesli with condensed milk according to the original recipe. Disadvantage: Although condensed milk is tolerated surprisingly well despite milk intolerance often it is available only with added sugar.

Sprouted cereal grains

These are particularly high in the vitamin E and B group, and generally have a strengthening effect.

How to sprout cereal grains:

1st day, evening: wash the grains on a screen under running water and put them in a bowl. Cover with water and keep at room temperature, close to the oven.

2nd day, morning: rinse the grains and spread to dry on a flat plate at room temperature, close to the oven. The same evening, put them back in the bowl and cover with water. Keep at room temperature, close to the oven.

3rd day, morning: rinse the grains and spread to dry on the plate. Evening: put the grains back in the bowl and cover with water. Keep at room temperature, close to the oven.

On the 4th day, the grains should have developed sprouts of 1–2 cm and are ready to eat.

The preparation of sprouted cereal grains is easier in the practical sprouting devices that are available in different sizes.

Sprouted cereal grains are suitable to prepare muesli but also as an addition to salads or raw vegetables.

Linomel muesli according to Dr. Johanna Budwig

1 teaspoon honey
2 tablespoons milk, gently warmed
1–2 tablespoons linseed oil
50–100 g low-fat quark
2–3 teaspoons Linomel flax seed/honey granulate, available from health-food stores)
150–200 g fresh seasonal fruit
1 tablespoon sunflower seeds or ground almonds or hazelnuts

Put 2–3 tablespoons of Linomel into a small dish, add the chopped fruits (if desired, enriched with softened raisins, sultanas or wine berries).
Mix honey, milk and flax seed oil with a mixer or whisk, gradually add the quark and stir the mixture into a smooth, thick cream.
Pour over the fruits and spread the sunflower seeds or ground nuts on top.

Raw vegetables and salads

Observe three considerations when preparing raw vegetables and salads:

1. Freshness and quality

For diet at hypertension and arteriosclerosis, for any other diet and for everyday nutrition, use only sun ripened, organically grown vegetables and salads. They are not only ideal for health but also have the best taste. Today the offer from organically run operations is very large, and organically grown vegetables are available even in supermarkets. But of course it is particularly suitable to use vegetables and salads from your own garden. Herbs and tomatoes can be grown even on a balcony. Choose young, tender leafy lettuces and root vegetables, not blanched, without any wilted leaves or rotting stalks. For a healing regime it is important to use only entirely fresh and high quality plants.

Prepare raw vegetables just before eating them and mix them with the dressing immediately. Letting them stand will markedly reduce the vitamin content of the chopped vegetables and salads.

2. Cleanliness

Vegetables grown organically without manure fertilisation contain no worm eggs. Nevertheless, all fresh plants must be cleaned thoroughly and carefully. Observe that water soluble substances such as vitamin C, vitamins of the B-group and minerals are leached out in water. Therefore, only wash directly under the tap set to shower.

3. Harmonious composition

Every salad dish should contain all three types of vegetables: root, fruit and leaf. Green leafy lettuce in particular is always part of a healing regime. The individual salads or raw vegetables should each have an appropriate dressing so that they are appetizing. Suitable dressings are listed in the table below.

A beautifully assembled salad in pleasing colours is agreeable to the eye and the palate, and stimulates the appetite. Small garnishes of herbs, radishes, young carrots or olives make the raw vegetable dish even more colourful and festive. The three kinds of vegetables should not be exceeded per meal for everyday use. Too much variety may impair digestion.

Cleaning leafy vegetables

For head lettuce, endives, romaine lettuce, iceberg lettuce and similar green leaf lettuces, cabbage and red cabbage, etc. separate the leaves and clean them individually and carefully under running water. Rinse several times and spin dry thoroughly.

Small-leaved salads such as lamb's lettuce and cut lettuce, spinach, dandelion, cress, rocket, radicchio and Brussels sprouts should be rinsed repeatedly in small portions and any hard stalks removed. Halve chicory/endive, remove outer leaves and rinse well.

Cleaning root vegetables

Celery, carrots, horseradish, radish, beetroot, kohlrabi, black salsify: clean with a brush under running water, peel and immediately grate or plane into the finished sauce. Mix well to preserve the vegetables' fresh colour.

Cleaning vegetable fruits

Wash tomatoes and cut them into wedges or slices. Peel cucumbers and cut them small or grate them. Organically grown young cucumbers are more nutritious if they have not been peeled.
Use only young, tender unpeeled courgettes for salads, wash them thoroughly and slice or julienne them. Green and yellow sweet pepper is less hot than the red variety. Wash, halve, remove seeds and cut small. Unfortunately, today almost all non-organic sweet peppers are from hydroponic production.
Separate cauliflower and broccoli into florets, and clean thoroughly under running water.
Wash stalk celery, peel it, and cut away hard parts.
Halve leeks and fennel, prepare and wash under the tap set to shower.
Bircher-Benner manual no. 4 contains essential instructions for cleaning and preparing raw food.

Salad dressings

Sparing use of table salt is particularly important for the diet for patients with hypertension and arteriosclerosis. Salad dressings need no salt and will still be highly aromatic.
Alternate the herbs often – this will avoid any boredom. Today, you can purchase fresh herbs of good quality almost all the year round. If not, use dried herbs.

Oil dressing

2 tablespoons oil (rapeseed, sunflower or olive oil from first cold pressing, thistle oil, walnut oil)
1 teaspoon fresh, cold pressed flax seed oil
1 teaspoon lemon juice or organic fruit vinegar
If tolerated, a little fresh garlic, pressed or finely ground
1 teaspoon fresh herbs (or knife tip dried herbs).

Mix all the ingredients and whisk the dressing until creamy. The dressing also is even tastier with a splash of soy sauce or Kelpamare.
This classic salad dressing is suited to all green salads (head lettuce, romaine lettuce, cress, etc.) and fruit salads (tomatoes, cucumbers etc.).

Quark dressing
If milk protein is permitted.

1 tablespoon lean quark
3 tablespoons butter milk
$1/2$ teaspoon lemon juice
fresh, finely chopped herbs

Whisk all ingredients thoroughly.

This dressing goes particularly well with root vegetables (carrots, celery, radishes, etc.).

Yoghurt dressing
If milk protein is permitted.

2–3 tablespoons yoghurt
a few drops of lemon juice
onion, grated
a little garlic, pressed
1 teaspoon fresh herbs (or 1 knife tip dried herbs)

Whisk all ingredients thoroughly.
A refreshing dressing with cress or spinach, with fruit salads (tomatoes, cucumbers) and with root vegetables (kohlrabi, horseradish, radishes).

Cream dressing
For stage–IV diet only

2 tablespoons sour cream
1 teaspoon lean quark
1 teaspoon lemon juice
very little pepper
1 teaspoon fresh herbs (or 1 knife tip dried herbs)

Whisk all ingredients thoroughly.

This dressing suits almost all root and fruit salads. For a change, you may replace lemon juice with orange juice, to give the raw food a new flavour. With celery root/celeriac, beetroot and chicory/endive salad, you can add a little freshly ground horseradish to this sauce for a very exciting flavour.

Lemon dressing
Much more nutritious than vinegar dressing

2 tablespoons fresh lemon juice
1 tablespoon agave syrup (Allos brand, available in health-food stores)
1 teaspoon olive oil
a little minced onion
1 teaspoon salad herbs mixture or Ysop

Mix all ingredients well.
This dressing goes well with all salads, particularly dark green leafy salads. In spring, add a few daisies to the green salad. They are very rich in nutrients and look pretty.

Orange dressing
1 small lemon
2 large oranges
1 tablespoon freshly ground coriander
1 piece fresh ginger
(for 2 dl sauce)

Press oranges and lemon and mix well. Add coriander and finely ground ginger. If you like your dressing slightly sweet (particularly good with carrots or beetroot), add 1 teaspoon thick agave juice (Allos).

The root vegetables should be marinated in the dressing for at least 3 hours. Before serving, you can dress the salad with a very small amount of olive oil.

Garlic dressing
1 garlic clove (in spring, 2 wild-onion leaves)
2 teaspoons thistle or sunflower oil
1 teaspoon flax seed oil
1 tablespoon apple vinegar
1 tablespoon unrefined sugar (Panela, Succanat)

Put the sugar in the vinegar overnight to dissolve it completely. Mix oil and vinegar well with a whisk; add the pressed garlic clove or finely cut wild onion leaves.

This dressing tastes great with vegetable-blossom salads such as broccoli, cauliflower or romanesco.

Peppermint dressing
2 tablespoons fresh lemon juice
1 tablespoon honey or agave syrup
1 tablespoon olive oil (optional)
lots of fresh peppermint leaves

Whisk liquid ingredients thoroughly. Chop the peppermint leaves and mix them in.

This scented, green dressing goes wonderfully with sugar peas and with finely cut romaine lettuce.

Nut dressing
2 tablespoons sour cream
1 tablespoon hazelnut or almond paste
1 teaspoon lemon juice
a touch of honey
1 pinch ginger
1 tablespoon coarsely chopped walnuts, hazelnuts or almonds

Whisk all ingredients thoroughly.

A pretty dressing for root vegetables. It also goes well with chopped Belgian endive. For variety, you may add a little finely sliced apple.

Almond- or sesame-puree dressing
1 tablespoon almond or sesame puree
3 tablespoons water
1 teaspoon lemon juice
a little garlic, pressed
1 teaspoon fresh herbs (or knife tip dried herbs)

Slowly stir sesame or almond puree with water until smooth, then add the other ingredients.

This tasty dressing goes very well with root vegetables.

Mayonnaise with wholegrain soy flour instead of egg
(for 6 – 8 portions)
2 tablespoons soy wholegrain flour
6 tablespoons water
2 dl oil

Mix soy wholegrain flour and water until smooth. Slowly add oil while constantly stirring with the whisk.
The mayonnaise can be kept in the fridge for a few days.

For 1 portion you need:
1 tablespoon mayonnaise
1 teaspoon lemon juice
a touch of mustard (optional)
1 teaspoon fresh herbs (or knife tip dried herbs)

Mix all ingredients well.
Mayonnaise is a popular dressing for

salads composed of field and root vegetables.

Sauerkraut salad
Sauerkraut is a very valuable raw vegetable, especially in winter. It is more easily digestible raw than cooked, and has a gallbladder-purging and disinfecting effect. An addition of shredded raw sauerkraut can improve taste and tolerability considerably. For a salad, sauerkraut is loosely separated and chopped, mixed with a few caraway seeds (or ground caraway), 3–4 chopped juniper berries, sliced onion, a julienned apple or a diced small fresh pineapple. Choose oil dressing as a dressing. This salad goes particularly well with corn salad and a raw-root vegetable.

Table to Choose Suitable Salad Dressings

Suggestions for dressings matching the salads and raw vegetables

head lettuce	uncut	oil dressing	chives, onion
cut lettuce	uncut	oil dressing	chives, onion
endive/chicory	cut in strips of 1 cm	oil dressing	onion, parsley
lamb's lettuce	uncut	oil dressing	onion, parsley
cress	uncut	yoghurt dressing	chives
spinach	cut strips of $1/2$ cm	yoghurt dressing	peppermint
cabbage lettuces: white cabbage, sauerkraut, Brussels sprouts, savoy cabbage	slice, cut into thin pieces	oil dressing or nut dressing	lovage, savory, thyme, caraway
tomatoes	slice or dice	oil dressing or yoghurt dressing	basil, thyme, oregano
cucumbers	slice	oil dressing	dill
fennel	finely cut with knife	cream dressing or oil dressing	dill, chives, parsley
sweet peppers	cut into fine strips	oil dressing or mayonnaise	chives
radish	slice or grate	quark dressing	chives, parsley
radishes	slice or cut finely	yoghurt dressing	chives, parsley
stalk celery	cut finely	oil dressing or almond-puree dressing	chives, thyme
courgettes	grate coarsely or slice	oil dressing or almond-puree dressing	dill, borage, basil
beets	grate finely	yoghurt or orange dressing	chives, lovage
Celery (celeriac)	grate finely	nut dressing	ginger
beetroot	grate finely	cream sauce	horseradish
cauliflower, broccoli	cut off florets, grate stems	garlic dressing	chives
Chicory/endive	cut in strips of 1 cm	cream sauce	tarragon, parsley
Jerusalem artichoke	grate	mayonnaise	marjoram, thyme
kohlrabi	slice or grate	yoghurt dressing or nut dressing	thyme, lovage
red cabbage	slice or cut finely	almond-puree dressing	some grated apple, caraway, lovage

Milk Types

Almond milk
This mild food provides vegetable protein and oil and is rich in valuable unsaturated plant oils. Stimulates mucous production and soothes.

1 tablespoon almond puree
1½ teaspoons honey
6 dl water

Add almond puree and honey to the water in the shaker and mix until smooth. You may add a fruit of your choice.

Almond milk of fresh almonds
Particularly easy to digest.

1½ tablespoons almonds, peeled (no bitter ones)
1 teaspoon honey
1½ dl water

Mix almonds, honey and water in the mixer. Strain if necessary.

Pine nut milk
Very rich in easily digestible vegetable oils and protein that protects the metabolism.

1½ tablespoons pine nuts, washed
1 teaspoon honey
1½ dl water

Prepare in the blender like almond milk.

Sesame milk
2 dl water (cold or warm)
1 level tablespoon sesame puree
1 teaspoon lemon juice
1 teaspoon honey

Put sesame puree, honey and lemon juice in the water and mix well.

Sesame cream
Like sesame milk, but with ⅓ as much water added. Replaces cream in cooked dishes and desserts.

Sesame frappé
Like sesame milk or sesame cream, with addition of fruit juice, apple juice, fruit concentrates.

Soy milk
1 cup soy beans
7 cups water
1 tablespoon fruit sugar

Wash and dry soy beans and grind them in an almond mill. Soak for 2 hours, then boil for 20 min. in the water used for soaking, stirring constantly. Strain. Add water until the viscosity of cow's milk is reached. Add fruit sugar and let cool. Soy milk is sold in tetra packs in the health-food store.

Plant fats, oils and butter

The Bircher kitchen uses only cold-pressed oils and almond purees and other nut spreads for raw food. Cooked food may also be prepared using small amounts of fresh butter, olive oil and unhardened vegetable fats. Olive oil may be heated up to 170 °C. Other plant oils with polyunsaturated fatty acids must never be heated, since the unsaturated fatty acids may turn into dangerous radicals.

Olive oil
Olive oil is often suitable for refining dishes.

Fresh butter
To enhance dishes for which olive oil is not suitable.

Vegetable margarine and food fats procured from health-food stores (Nussella,

Becel and Olim in Switzerland; Vitaquell and Eden in Germany) are vegetable fat emulsions of naturally firm (i.e. unhardened) fats such as coconut oil or palm seed oil mixed with the maximum proportion of liquid oils and seed oils, particularly olive oil. Margarines with hydrogenated fats should never be used.

Nut spread and almond puree
These plant fats have a very fine, nutty flavour. They can be used variously as bland food or to replace fresh butter. They should never be heated. Olive oil is suitable for vegetables, potatoes, rice, pasta.

Cold-pressed sunflower oil, corn seed oil, thistle oil, cold-pressed olive oil
Organic and carefully treated, rich in highly unsaturated fatty acids, these fats are more easily digestible for most people than butter. Apart from olive oil, which contains no polyunsaturated fatty acids (only monounsaturated ones), vegetable oils must never be heated, since this may lead to the formation of dangerous carcinogenic radicals.

Fresh cold-pressed flax seed oil contains approx. 60 % omega-3 fatty acids. The ratio of omega-6 fatty acids to omega-3 fatty acids must be at least 1:5 (1:2 or 1:3 is better). If the flax seed oil is fresh, it does not have a very strong taste and can be added to Birchermuesli and salad dressings every day. Mixed with a little lemon juice, flax seed oil enhances certain raw vegetables and Linomel muesli (see recipe page 103). Flax seed oil should be a part of daily diet. It is very digestible and can be conveniently consumed straight from the spoon (2 tablespoons twice a day). Do not leave the oil exposed to the air, but keep it tightly closed in the refrigerator. The addition of lemon juice protects the oil from oxidation. Flax seed oil with lemon juice and a little dill is particularly suitable for fresh avocados.

Gentle cooking and steaming/sautéing

Today hardly any housewife or working woman will want to do without her pressure cooker. This appliance is time-saving and far more healthful than other methods. Who would want to forgo these advantages?

The pressure cooker works especially well for soups and is useful for almost every other recipe. The cooking time is only $1/3$ to $1/4$ of the normal cooking time.

Many vegetable and potato recipes can also be steamed gently and very quickly in the pressure cooker, resulting in dishes that retain their colour, flavour, vitamins and nutrients. If you like your vegetables firmer (al dente), the cooking time of vegetables (except potatoes) can be reduced to taste, even with conventional steaming.
For cereal dishes, we recommend using the steamer for grains with long cooking times (e.g. coarse corn, wholegrain rice), but not for pasta products.

Soups

The recipes are for 1 person.

The following soup and vegetable recipes use a lot of vegetable broth. In a small household, it is inconvenient to make fresh vegetable broth every day. Instead, you may use ordinary water and salt-free vegetable bouillon cubes. The yeast extracts from the health-food store are very rich in vitamin B and in important glutathione and lecithin. However, they also contain sea salt and should therefore be used only sparingly or, in cases of hypertension, not at all.
Cream enriches soups and vegetables, but olive oil can usually be used instead.
In case of wheat allergy, the wholegrain

flour in the recipes should be replaced by rice, millet or oat flour.

Vegetable broth
Unlike other recipes in this book, this recipe is for 4 persons:

1 tablespoon olive oil
1 onion
2 carrots
1 small stalk of celery (150 g)
cabbage, chard leaves
1 leek stalk
3–4 l water
½ bay leaf
1 pinch rock salt
lovage, basil or other herbs, dried or preferably fresh

Halve the onion, keeping the brown peel, and brown the cut area briefly in olive oil at low heat. Chop the vegetables, add them and cook for at least 15 min. covered at low heat. Add water and cook for 2 hours at low heat. Season to taste (except for salt).

Vegetable bouillon
3 dl vegetable broth
a little yeast extract (health-food store) or Kelpamare (optional)
10 g nut spread or olive oil
parsley, chives, freshly chopped herbs

Prepare the vegetable broth according to the above recipe and add to nut spread, olive oil and herbs.

Rice soup, clear
½ tablespoon olive oil
a little chopped onion
1 small carrot
a little celery root (celeriac) and leek
1 tablespoon rice
6 dl vegetable broth
chives

Sauté onion with finely cut vegetables and rice. Add hot vegetable broth and cook for 15–20 minutes. Prepare with finely cut chives and olive oil.

Rice soup, thickened
½ tablespoon olive oil
a little celery root (celeriac) and leek
1 small carrot
1 tablespoon rice
½ tablespoon wholegrain flour
6 dl vegetable broth or water
lovage, parsley, basil, marjoram
a little soya sauce (optional)
½ tablespoon sesame cream (see recipe page 109)
chives

Sauté the chopped vegetables in oil. Sprinkle with wholegrain flour, pour on vegetable broth and cook for 30 minutes. Season with soya sauce and herbs. Place cream and finely cut chives in the soup bowl and serve the soup over them.

Herbal soup
1 tablespoon wholegrain flour
1 dl water
5 dl vegetable broth
1 tablespoon cream
5 g butter, olive oil or nut spread (optional)
lovage, basil, tarragon, marjoram, chives, nutmeg or caraway (optional)

Stir wholegrain flour into cold water and add to the boiling vegetable broth. Cook for 15 minutes. Season with the herbs. Add cream (or optional butter, olive oil, or nut spread) to the soup bowl, add the soup and whisk.

Oat cream soup
½ tablespoon olive oil
2 tablespoons fine or coarse oat flakes
6 dl vegetable broth
a little celery root (celeriac)
1 tablespoon sesame cream
(see recipe page 109)
optional: miso, chives, nutmeg or caraway

Briefly sauté oat flakes. Add vegetable broth and celery (celeriac). Slightly cook oat flakes for 10 minutes (coarse ones for at least 20 minutes). Season to taste. Place sesame cream and chives in the soup bowl and add the pureed soup.

Oat groat soup
½ tablespoon olive oil
2 tablespoons oat groats
some chopped onion
7 dl water or vegetable broth
1 dl milk
a little diced celery root (celeriac)
1 pinch sea salt or some miso
1 tablespoon cream (optional)
chives, parsley, marjoram or borage

Sauté onion and groats with or without olive oil. Add vegetable broth, milk and celery root (celeriac) and cook for 45–60 minutes. Season to taste with sea salt or miso. Place cream and herbs in the soup bowl and add the soup.

Semolina soup
1 tablespoon semolina
5 dl vegetable broth
1 tablespoon sesame cream (see recipe page 109)
5 g fresh butter, or ½ tablespoon olive oil or nut spread
1 pinch rock salt
caraway, nutmeg (optional)
lovage, basil, marjoram, parsley, chives

Stir semolina into the boiling vegetable broth, add pinch of salt and caraway, and cook for ½ hour. Season to taste with herbs. Place sesame cream and butter (or olive oil or nut spread) in the soup bowl and add the soup.

Tomato soup
½ tablespoon olive oil
a little onion, celery root (celeriac) and leek
1 small carrot
1 garlic clove
1 tomato
1 tablespoon wholegrain flour
6 dl vegetable broth
1 pinch rock salt
a touch of mild mustard (optional)
1 pinch fruit sugar (or Sucanat)
rosemary, oregano
5 g olive oil or nut spread
1 tablespoon sesame cream (see recipe page 109)
chives

Sauté vegetables cut small with or without olive oil, then add the tomato. Sprinkle with wholegrain flour and pour the vegetable broth into the mixture. Cook for ½ hour then strain. Add spices and mustard (optional). Place olive oil or nut spread and sesame cream in the soup bowl and add the finished soup. Sprinkle with finely cut chives. If desired, add 1 tablespoon rice to the soup or sprinkle with fat-free toasted wholegrain bread cubes.

Summer tomato soup
4 ripe tomatoes
1 pinch fruit sugar
1 pinch rock salt
¼ dl cream

Dice the tomatoes, cook briefly, season and strain. Add cream and serve the soup lukewarm or cold.

Vegetable soups (carrots, spinach, broccoli)
½ tablespoon olive oil
a little chopped onion
1½ tablespoons wholegrain flour
1 pinch rock salt
5 dl vegetable broth
1 dl water or, if permitted, milk
1 tablespoon sesame cream (see recipe page 109)
Vegetables: 1 carrot, cut small, or 1 small cup of spinach, pureed or finely chopped, broccoli finely chopped (cook some of the flowers separately and set them aside).

Sauté onion and carrots or broccoli with or without olive oil. Sprinkle with wholegrain flour and sauté them together briefly. Pour in vegetable broth and water (or milk) and cook for 20–40 minutes. For the spinach soup, add the spinach last and remove from heat. Pour the soup over the sesame cream in the soup bowl. For the broccoli soup, add the flowers previously set aside.

Seasoning the vegetable soups:

For carrot soup, use celery leaves or lovage, rosemary or marjoram, 1 teaspoon caraway.
For spinach soup, use peppermint leaves, parsley, chives, pinch of nutmeg.
For broccoli soup, use a little basil, parsley, chives, tarragon.

Chervil soup
½ tablespoon olive oil
a little onion
1 medium-sized potato, chopped in cubes
½ tablespoon wholegrain flour
5 dl vegetable broth
1 pinch rock salt
1 tablespoon chervil, chopped
1 tablespoon cream

Sauté the onion slightly with or without olive oil. Add potato, sprinkle with wholegrain flour and add vegetable broth and a pinch of salt. Cook for ½ hour and strain. Put chervil and cream in the soup bowl and add the soup.

Potato soup
½ leek, cut into thin strips
½ carrot, sliced
½ tablespoon wholegrain flour
5 dl vegetable broth
1 medium-sized potato, diced
1 pinch rock salt
basil, marjoram
1 tablespoon cream

Sauté the leek and carrot in a little vegetable broth. Sprinkle with wholegrain flour and add the vegetable broth. Add potato and cook until soft. Season. Put basil, marjoram and optional cream in the soup bowl and add the finished soup.

Minestrone
½ tablespoon olive oil
2 tablespoon leek
a little onion, finely chopped
a few celery leaves
½ plateful beet greens
7 dl water or vegetable broth
1 tablespoon lovage or thyme
½ garlic clove, pressed
basil, parsley, chives
1 pinch rock salt
15 g pasta or rice
5 g butter or nut spread

Finely chop onion, leek, celery leaves and beet greens and sauté them slowly. Add vegetable broth, season and cook for ½ hour. Add pasta or rice and cook another 15–20 minutes. To enrich, add cream or nut spread.

Vegetables

Spinach, chopped
¼ l vegetable broth
200 g spinach (remove thick stems)
¼ garlic clove, pressed
1 pinch rock salt
peppermint leaves, sage
1 cup raw spinach
little optional nut spread or olive oil

Briefly cook spinach in the vegetable broth and drain, then finely cut, chop or blend. Return spinach to the pan and heat. Add garlic, salt and herbs. Chop, finely cut or blend the raw spinach and add to the cooked spinach (with a little optional olive oil or nut butter) before serving.

Spinach, whole leaves (and stems)
300 g spinach (remove thick stems, briefly boil the coarser winter spinach if required)
1 tablespoon pine nuts
1 tablespoon raisins (optional)
1 pinch rock salt
peppermint leaves, sage, parsley
optional: olive oil or nut spread

Steam spinach uncovered over low heat with very little water. Add pine nuts, spices and optional raisins and briefly continue cooking. Add olive oil or nut spread if desired.

Lettuce
1 romaine lettuce
1 l water
a little chopped onion
1 dl vegetable broth
1 pinch rock salt

Halve the romaine lettuce, boil until semi-soft then drain. Reassemble the lettuce and place in an oven-proof mould. Lightly sauté the onion without vegetable fat and place it over the lettuce. Add vegetable broth and a pinch of rock salt and cook in the oven for 30–40 min.

Endive/chicory
1 large endive head

Prepare just like romaine lettuce.

Sautéed chicory/endive

2 heads chicory/endive
½ tablespoon olive oil
3 tablespoons vegetable broth
1 pinch rock salt
marjoram, thyme
a little olive oil or nut spread

Halve the chicory/endive and layer the leaves in the pan. Add heated olive oil and vegetable broth to the chicory/endive, season and cook covered over low heat for ½ hour. At the end, spread melted nut spread or olive oil on the prepared vegetables.

Chard with béchamel sauce
3 chard stems
½ dl vegetable broth
a little lemon juice or 1 tablespoon almond puree
1 pinch rock salt
tarragon, parsley and chives
béchamel sauce (see recipe page 124)

Cut the chard leaves into pieces of 3 cm, cook covered over low heat for ½ to ¾ hour until soft with the vegetable broth and lemon juice (or almond puree). Season to taste and mix the fresh vegetables with béchamel sauce.

Celery stalks
3–4 stalks celery
½ onion, chopped
a little apple, finely chopped
1 dl vegetable broth
1 teaspoon almond puree
1 pinch rock salt or a little soya
celery greens

Cut the celery stalk into pieces 8 cm long and place in a pan. Briefly sauté the onion and apple without fat and spread on the celery. Add vegetable broth and cook over low heat for ½ to ¾ hour. Add almond puree once it has cooled. Season.

Baked fennel with cream cheese
(Only for stage IV diet)
1 large or 2 small fennel plants
1 pinch rock salt
pepper
several drops of lemon juice
10 g cream cheese

Quarter the fennel and steam it until semi-soft. Pull apart the individual layers of the fennel bulb and place them in an oven-proof mould. Drizzle with lemon juice, then add salt and pepper. Stir the cream cheese with 2 tablespoons of fennel stock and spread on the vegetables. Bake in hot oven.

Vegetable curry
1 tablespoon olive oil
1 spring onion
200 g vegetables (e.g. leeks, carrots, courgettes, asparagus)
$1/2$ teaspoon wholegrain flour
1 knife tip (to taste) curry powder
$1/2$ teaspoon vegetable broth
$1/2$ orange
1 teaspoon sultanas
1 pinch whole sugar (or Sucanat)
1 pinch rock salt, pepper

Cut the spring onion into fine rings and cook in slightly heated oil. Sprinkle on flour and curry powder and add the vegetable broth. Add the cut small vegetables and cook covered for approx. 15 minutes. Set aside two or three wedges of the orange, squeeze the rest and place the sultanas in the juice. When the vegetables are soft, add the sultanas and orange juice, heat the mixture and season with sugar, salt and pepper. Serve and spread the orange wedges on top.

Cooked carrots
3–4 carrots
1 dl vegetable broth
1 teaspoon almond puree
1 pinch each fruit sugar and sea salt
marjoram, thyme, rosemary, parsley

Cut the carrots in strips or rounds and cook in the vegetable broth for 30–45 min. Season. When the mixture has cooled somewhat, stir in the almond puree and sprinkle with chopped parsley.

Peas and carrots
100 g fresh peas, shelled
1 dl vegetable broth
marjoram, thyme, lovage
parsley, chives
150 g sliced carrots, prepared according to the above recipe for cooked carrots

Cook peas in the vegetable broth until soft. Season. Mix carrots and peas, or serve separately.

Peas, French style
¼ head of lettuce or romaine lettuce
150–200 g peas, shelled
1 dl vegetable broth
1 pinch rock salt
parsley, chives marjoram, thyme, lovage
10 g nut spread
1 teaspoon wholegrain flour

Sauté the lettuce or romaine lettuce cut into fine strips with the peas in the vegetable broth over very low heat until soft. Season. Mix nut spread with wholegrain flour, add and boil briefly.

Cooked sugar peas (snow peas)
200 g snow peas
1 dl vegetable broth
1 pinch rock salt
1 pinch sugar (Succanat)
a little parsley or lovage
chives, marjoram, thyme
olive oil or nut spread

Cook sugar peas and herbs covered in the vegetable broth for $1/2$ to $3/4$ hour. Season and add olive oil or nut spread when serving.

Green beans with tomatoes
250 g beans
a little garlic
savoury, parsley
1–2 tomatoes
1 pinch rock salt
some caraway, marjoram, lovage

Sauté the beans, finely diced tomatoes and herbs for approx. 1 hour. Add some water if necessary. Season to taste.

Steamed celery root (celeriac)
½ celery
1 dl vegetable broth
1 pinch rock salt

some lemon juice, marjoram
1 teaspoon almond puree
very thin slices of apple, nuts

Pour vegetable broth over the julienned celery root (celeriac) and cook until soft, $1/2$ to $3/4$ hour. Season. Add apple slices. To refine, add almond puree once the mixture has cooled down. Sprinkle with chopped nuts.

Celery with béchamel sauce
Prepare 1 small celery stalk as described above and mix with béchamel sauce (see recipe page 124).

Beetroots
Cut off the root tips and leaves to approx. 2 cm and wash thoroughly without damaging the skin.

350 g beetroots
1 dl vegetable broth
1 pinch each fruit sugar and
1 pinch rock salt
$1/4$ laurel leaf, lovage, caraway, nutmeg
touch of garlic, parsley, lemon juice, lemon balm
1 tablespoon wholegrain flour, mixed cold
1 tablespoon almond puree

Cook the beetroots soft in the pressure cooker for approx. 25 min. Peel and cut into thin slices. Mix thoroughly with the herbs and spices in the vegetable broth and cook over low heat for 15 min. To bind, stir in the wholegrain flour and finally, once it has cooled somewhat, add the almond puree.

Jerusalem artichoke
250 g Jerusalem artichoke
a little vegetable broth
1 pinch rock salt
basil
1 teaspoon almond puree

Cook the Jerusalem artichoke like jacket potatoes (see recipe page 119). Peel, slice and cook until soft in the vegetable broth. Once it has cooled somewhat, season and add the almond puree to refine.
You can also prepare the Jerusalem artichoke with béchamel sauce (see recipe page 124).

Stewed tomatoes
4–5 tomatoes
$1/2$ tablespoon olive oil
$1/2$ onion
1 teaspoon fruit sugar
1 pinch rock salt
touch of garlic, rosemary, marjoram, basil
1 tablespoon corn starch (optional)
parsley or chives or dill

Slightly brown onion and fruit sugar in olive oil in the pan. Douse the tomatoes with boiling water then peel them, cut them into pieces, add them to the onions and cook the mixture until it has thickened a little. Add garlic and spices and finish cooking (add corn starch to thicken). Sprinkle plenty of chopped parsley or other herbs on the prepared tomatoes.

Steamed tomatoes
2–3 tomatoes
1 tablespoon olive oil
$1/4$ onion, chopped
a pinch of herbes de Provence (basil, rosemary, thyme, sage, parsley)

Sauté the onion without fat. Put the halved tomatoes on a greased tray or oven-proof mould. Rub olive oil on each tomato half, and spread the sautéed onion and herbs on it. Cook briefly in the oven.
Some tomatoes may be minced or very finely chopped, blended with cream, reheated briefly and spread over the prepared tomato.

Stuffed tomatoes
2–3 tomatoes
1 teaspoon rice per tomato
1 pinch rock salt

olive oil or nut spread
a little onion and garlic
rosemary, marjoram, thyme, basil
bay leaf, nutmeg
vegetable broth (optional)

Cut out the top of the tomatoes and hollow out the core. Chop the tomato pulp and mix with 1 teaspoon uncooked rice and the herbs and spices. Fill in the core with the mixture, add olive oil or nut spread, and replace the tops of the tomatoes. Bake in the oven at a bottom heat of 160° for 20–30 min.

Tomatoes à la provençale
2 tomatoes
1 tablespoon olive oil
1 tablespoon chopped parsley
1 tablespoon breadcrumbs

Halve tomatoes and place on a tray. Rub olive oil on them, mix breadcrumbs and parsley and spread on the tomatoes with a spoon. Bake in the oven for 15 min.

Courgettes with tomatoes
1/2 onion, chopped
300 g courgette
50 g tomato
garlic, rosemary, marjoram, thyme, basil
parsley, chives, dill
maize flour (optional)
1 teaspoon almond puree

Sauté the onion without fat. Dice the courgettes; peel and dice the tomatoes. Add the vegetables to the onions and cook until soft. Season. If there is too much liquid, add maize flour and, once it has cooled somewhat, 1 teaspoon almond puree before serving.

Sweet peppers (green, yellow, red)
These are very suitable as addition to other dishes.

150–200 g sweet peppers
1/2 tablespoon olive oil
1/2 onion, chopped
1 pinch rock salt
garlic, rosemary, marjoram, thyme, basil, parsley

Cut the sweet peppers in strips and sauté them in olive oil with the onion, herbs and spices in a covered pan for at least 1/2 hour.

Ratatouille
50 g sweet peppers
100 g courgette
50 g aubergine
1 tomato
1/2 onion, chopped
a little garlic
1 tablespoon olive oil
1 pinch rock salt
rosemary, marjoram, thyme, basil, parsley

Chop the sweet peppers, courgettes, aubergines and tomato (peeled). Sauté onion and garlic in plant fat, add vegetables and cook covered for 1 hour. Season. If there is too much sauce, let it thicken while uncovered.

Artichokes
1 artichoke
3/4 l water
1 tablespoon lemon juice
1 pinch rock salt

Cut off the stalks close to the artichokes. Remove the bottommost hard leaves and remove the tips. Halve and cut out the heart; wash under running water and rub the cut surface with lemon juice. Bring water to the boil, add lemon juice and rock salt and cook the artichoke until soft for approx. 3/4 h. Drain and serve the artichoke on a warm platter covered with a serviette. Serve with yoghurt sauce (see recipe page 105).

Asparagus
1/2 bunch of asparagus
1 l water

1 pinch rock salt
nut spread

Wash the asparagus and peel the stalks thoroughly. Green asparagus can be left almost whole. Cook the asparagus in boiling water until soft for 20–30 min. (green asparagus take much less time), remove with a perforated spoon and serve on a platter covered with a serviette. Pour liquid nut spread over the dish.
As a variation, serve with vinaigrette sauce (see recipe page 126).

Cauliflower or broccoli
1 small cauliflower or broccoli (250 g)
1 teaspoon olive oil
1 garlic clove
1 dl vegetable broth
1 pinch rock salt, pepper
pine nuts or almond slices

Cut off the leaves and stalk below the florets. Peel the stalk and cut into larger pieces; divide the flower into florets. Lightly brown the chopped garlic clove in olive oil, add the cauliflower or broccoli and sauté briefly. Douse with the vegetable broth and then cook for approx. 5 minutes. Season with salt and pepper. Briefly roast pine nuts or sliced almond without fat in a pan and spread on the vegetables.

Kohlrabi with herbs
1 kohlrabi
1 dl vegetable broth
1 tablespoon tender kohlrabi leaves, chopped
Béchamel sauce (see recipe page 124)

Cut kohlrabi into 4 pieces then into fine slices. Cook covered in the vegetable broth for $1/2$–$3/4$ hour. Add the kohlrabi leaves and cream before serving.
Mix the béchamel sauce with chopped herbs and pour over the cooked kohlrabi.

Corn on the cob
(Chew very well, otherwise hard to digest.)

1 corn cob
1–2 tablespoons quark or 10 g fresh butter

Use only corn cobs with tender and milky kernels. Remove the husks and strings. Cook the corn cob soft in boiling water for 10–20 min. and serve it on a hot plate. Blend fresh butter or quark with herbs and serve with the corn.

Salads of cooked vegetables

These salads are not considered raw food.

Carrots, celery, beetroot, beans, cauliflower, broccoli, courgettes, beet greens and chard are particularly suitable for these salads.
The vegetables are cooked until soft in vegetable broth or water, drained and cut small (diced, sliced, florets, strips). Serve with salad dressing or with vinaigrette or mayonnaise. Use onions and chopped herbs to enhance.

Potato salad
200 g potatoes
$1/2$ dl vegetable broth
1 tablespoon mayonnaise (see recipe page 126)
$1/2$ tablespoon chopped onions
borage, chives, parsley, lemon balm, marjoram, thyme, dill

Cook the potatoes until soft in the pressure cooker, peel while hot, and slice. Pour the heated vegetable broth over them and let stand for a bit, then mix in the mayonnaise. Season with onions and herbs.

Potato salad with cucumbers
1 large potato
$1/4$ cucumber

2 tablespoon yoghurt sauce (see recipe page 105)
½ garlic clove
dill or borage, chives, parsley, onion

Prepare the potato as described above. Grate the peeled cucumber with a coarse grater and add to the potato. Mix with yoghurt sauce and season with onions and herbs.
Rub the salad bowl with the garlic clove before serving.

Salade niçoise
1 boiled potato
1 small tomato
a few radishes
several cucumber slices
1 tablespoon olive oil
½ tablespoon lemon juice
1 pinch rock salt
parsley, chives or dill, lemon balm, borage
a few leaves of head lettuce

Slice the potato, tomato and radish and add a salad dressing of oil, lemon juice, a pinch of rock salt and herbs. Just before serving cut the leaves of head lettuce into broad strips and mix with the salad or prepare the salad on the head-lettuce leaves.

Rice salad
50 g rice
2 dl water
2 tablespoons quark sauce (see recipe page 105)
½ tablespoon chopped onions
¼ tomato
chives, parsley or basil
a few salad leaves

Cook the rice in water, rinse it briefly and let it cool. Add the onion, finely diced tomato and herbs to the quark sauce. Mix the rice with the dressing and prepare on salad leaves.

Celery root (celeriac) salad with soy mayonnaise
½ small celery root (celeriac)
½–1 tablespoon lemon juice
2 walnuts
¼ apple (optional)
1 pinch rock salt
1 tablespoon soy mayonnaise (see recipe page 106)

Cut the raw celery root into match-thin strips or grate it. Add lemon juice to prevent browning. Add the coarsely chopped walnuts and the grated apple and mix with the mayonnaise.

Vegetable aspics
2½ dl vegetable broth
2 g agar-agar
drops of lemon juice
some Kelpamare
fresh slices of cucumber
cubes of tomato
cooked broccoli flowers
cooked peas
cooked beans, finely chopped

Agar-agar is a plant-based gelatine powder that is used for vegetable and fruit aspics, sauces and puddings, etc. instead of animal gelatine.
Add agar-agar powder to the lukewarm vegetable broth and heat slowly until the gelling agent is thoroughly dissolved. Season with lemon juice and Kelpamare. Pour a little aspic into the rinsed moulds and let it harden. Garnish with vegetable slices, add more aspic, let it harden and repeat until the moulds are filled.
Turn over the cooled aspics and serve on salad leaves.

Potato dishes

Potatoes in their skins
2–4 small potatoes
water

Brush and wash potatoes. Fill pan with steamer insert or wire screen with water up to the insert, add potatoes, cover and cook for 30 to 40 minutes (8–10 minutes in the pressure cooker).

Baked potatoes
3–4 small potatoes
1 tablespoon olive oil
nut spread

Brush and wash the potatoes. On the top, score the peel 3–4 times, brush with oil and bake them on a sheet with baking foil at medium heat for 30–40 min. Put a dab of nut spread on each of the cooked potatoes.

Quark potatoes
3–4 small potatoes
50 g low-fat quark
1–2 tablespoons milk or cream
chives or caraway or marjoram
1 pinch rock salt

Make a shallow cut into the top of the potatoes and prepare them as for baked potatoes. For the stuffing, stir quark with milk or cream until smooth and add seasonings. Use a spoon to spread into the shallow cut of the baked potatoes or apply with a piping bag.

Caraway potatoes
2–3 medium-sized, longish narrow potatoes
1 teaspoon caraway
1 pinch rock salt
1 tablespoon olive oil

Wash and clean the potatoes and cut them in half crosswise. Brush olive oil on the cuts. Sprinkle caraway and a pinch of salt on the cut side of the potatoes. Bake at medium heat for ¾ hour.

Bouillon potatoes
250 g potatoes
1–2 dl vegetable broth
1 pinch rock salt
lovage, thyme
1 tablespoon olive oil or 10 g nut spread

Wash potatoes, peel, halve or cut into pieces and cook until soft in the vegetable broth with the salt and spices. Spread olive oil or nut spread on the prepared potatoes.

Creamed potatoes
200 g potatoes
onion, chopped
1 dl vegetable broth
1 pinch rock salt
½ dl cream
thyme, nutmeg, parsley

Peel, slice and briefly sauté potatoes and onion without fat. Cook until soft with the vegetable broth and spices. Add cream before serving. Sprinkle the prepared potatoes with chopped parsley.

Potatoes with tomatoes
200 g potatoes
½ small onion
1 dl vegetable broth
1 small tomato
1 pinch rock salt
1 tablespoon sesame cream (see recipe page 109)
marjoram, rosemary or thyme

Briefly sauté the chopped onion and peeled, sliced potatoes without fat, then cook them in the vegetable broth until semi-soft. Cut the peeled tomato into wedges, add and finish cooking. Season. Add the sesame cream before serving.

Mashed potatoes
4 potatoes
dried tomatoes
olive oil or nut spread

Wash, peel, quarter and steam the potatoes until soft. Rice the potatoes onto a warm plate. Add olive oil or nut spread and garnish with minced dried tomatoes.

Potato puree
4 potatoes
1 dl milk
nutmeg
1 tablespoon olive oil
1 pinch rock salt
finely chopped marjoram and caraway
garlic
dried tomatoes

Peel and slice the potatoes and steam them until soft. Strain through the potato ricer. Heat milk, add the potato mash, stir until smooth and season. Add cream if desired. Serve on a hot platter, garnished with minced dried tomatoes.

Roast potatoes
2 small potatoes
enough water for steaming
1 pinch rock salt
1 dl vegetable broth
1–2 tablespoons sesame cream (see recipe page 109) or nut spread
nutmeg, thyme, parsley

Peel and halve potatoes and steam them until semi-soft. Put them on an oven-proof platter with the cut side down. Cover with vegetable broth. Season and roast in the oven until the liquid has thickened. Add cream or nut spread and continue roasting until the potatoes are lightly browned. Serve with the cut side facing up and sprinkle with chopped parsley.

Potato slices with spinach
1 large potato
1 dl vegetable broth
1 pinch rock salt
100 g spinach
some olive oil or nut spread
garlic, parsley, chives
peppermint, sage or nutmeg (optional)

Cut the peeled potato lengthwise into slices 1 cm thick and cook carefully until soft. Place on a buttered tray. Prepare the spinach like leaf spinach (see recipe page 114), season and distribute over the potatoes. Apply nut spread or olive oil. Bake briefly in the oven.

Potato goulash
1 onion
1 large potato
1 green sweet pepper
1–2 dl water
1 pinch rock salt
marjoram, thyme, rosemary, parsley

Finely dice the onion and potato, julienne the sweet pepper and cover with water in a pan. Cook until soft, approx. 15 minutes. Season well and serve.

Ayurveda potatoes
(An attractive, aromatic dish that yields 3–4 helpings)

5 large potatoes
½ soy drink
1 package of soy crème (substitute for crème fraîche)
1 bunch each of fresh dill, fresh chives and fresh parsley
juice of ½ lemon
1–2 teaspoons turmeric
½ teaspoon curry
soy sauce

Cut the cleaned potatoes into thick slices and cook them for approx. 5 minutes. In the meantime, slowly heat the soy drink in a pan, mixed with the soy crème (do not boil). Stir in turmeric and curry to taste and season with soy sauce. Put the potato slices in the sauce and simmer for approx. 10 minutes. Sprinkle the fresh, finely chopped herbs on the potatoes and serve at once.

Cereal Dishes

Japanese rice
80 g wholegrain rice
1½–2 dl vegetable bouillon
1 pinch rock salt
1 tablespoon olive oil
1 small peeled onion studded with clove and bay leaf

Put the rice in the cooking bouillon with the studded onion and boil for 40 minutes. Let cool and remove the onion. Reheat the rice in the oven and top with olive oil or nut spread before serving.

Risotto
80 g wholegrain rice
1 tablespoon chopped onion
2 dl vegetable broth or water
1 pinch rock salt
dried mushrooms
fresh herbs to taste
rosemary
1 tablespoon olive oil or nut spread
1 tablespoon of grated Parmesan cheese

Sauté the rice with the onion until the rice is translucent. Add the vegetable broth or hot water and cook until al dente (30–40 minutes). Add the finely chopped, dried mushrooms and herbs and cook briefly together. Before serving, mix in olive oil or nut spread and grated Parmesan cheese with a fork.

Saffron rice
Prepare like risotto. Dissolve a knife tip of saffron powder in a little bouillon and add to rice.

Riz creole with vegetables
80 g wholegrain rice
1 tablespoon diced vegetables (leeks, celery root (celeriac), carrots)
2 dl vegetable broth
1 pinch rock salt
bay leaf, cloves, nutmeg (optional)
freshly chopped herbs to taste

Briefly sauté rice and vegetables, add hot vegetable broth and spices and cook for 30–45 min.

Tomato rice
80 g wholegrain rice
1 tablespoon chopped onion
a little garlic, pressed
1 large tomato
approx. 1 dl vegetable broth
1 pinch rock salt
rosemary, marjoram, nutmeg
optional basil
1 tablespoon olive oil

Sauté onion, garlic and rice until the rice is translucent. Add peeled, diced tomato. Add vegetable broth and spices and cook for 30–45 min. Add olive oil before serving.

Rice with courgettes
80 g wholegrain rice
1 tablespoon onion, chopped
150 g courgettes
1 pinch rock salt
1½ dl vegetable broth or water
freshly chopped dill
1 tablespoon olive oil or nut spread

Dice the courgettes. Prepare dish as for tomato rice (see above).

Rice with spinach
80 g wholegrain rice
100 g spinach
some onion, chopped
2 dl vegetable broth or water
1 pinch rock salt
nutmeg and peppermint
10 g fresh butter, plant margarine or nut spread

Cut spinach coarsely. Prepare dish as for tomato rice (see above).

Risi bisi (rice with peas)
80 g wholegrain rice
150 g tender peas, shelled

some onion, chopped
1 pinch each of fruit sugar and rock salt
½ dl vegetable broth
1½–2 dl water
1 tablespoon olive oil or nut spread
parsley

Sauté onion with fruit sugar and a pinch of salt. Add the peas and cook briefly, then add vegetable broth and cook the peas until soft. Prepare risotto (according to the above recipe) in a separate pan. Add the peas to the cooked risotto. Before serving, top the prepared rice with olive oil or nut spread and chopped parsley.

Rice gratin with tomatoes
80 g wholegrain rice
2 small tomatoes
some onion, chopped
2 tablespoons vegetables (leek, celery root (celeriac), carrots)
1½ dl vegetable broth
1 pinch rock salt
parsley, lovage
½ tablespoon olive oil

Briefly sauté onion and very finely diced vegetables, add the rice and continue cooking until translucent. Douse in hot vegetable broth, season and cook for 30–45 min. Put the finished rice and the sliced tomatoes into an oven-proof mould in layers, top with dabs of butter or brush on olive oil, and bake in the oven for 10 min.

Indian rice dish
80 g wholegrain rice
2 dl vegetable broth
1 pinch rock salt
1 small banana
1 small apple
1 tablespoon raisins
1 teaspoon sunflower seeds
1 teaspoon sesame seeds
saffron, curry, fresh ginger root

Cook rice with vegetable broth and 1 pinch of rock salt until not quite soft (approx. 30–40 minutes). Mix the sliced banana, the peeled and sliced apple, and the raisins into the rice and continue boiling for 5–10 min. Season with saffron, curry and ginger root to taste. Sprinkle with sunflower seeds and lightly dry-roasted (without fat) sesame seeds.

Semolina mash
50 g semolina
3 dl milk
2 dl water
1 tablespoon sesame cream (see recipe page 109)
1 tablespoon each of fruit sugar and cinnamon

Stir semolina into the boiling liquid and cook for 15–20 min. Sprinkle the sesame cream and fruit sugar mixed with cinnamon onto the prepared semolina mash.

Polenta
50 g maize semolina, medium fine
3 dl water
nutmeg
1 pinch rock salt
½ tablespoon olive oil

Boil water and stir in the maize. Boil for 5 min. over low heat, stirring frequently. Season and continue boiling for 45–60 min. over low heat. You may also add onion slices sautéed without fat.

Millet risotto
50 g millet
1 tablespoon chopped onion
1½ dl vegetable broth
½ onion
1 pinch rock salt

Sauté onion and hot-rinsed millet until glazed, add the hot vegetable broth and salt, and cook for 20 min. Before serving, top with julienned or sliced onion sautéed without fat.

Millet risotto with vegetables
40 g millet
1 tablespoon chopped onion
2 tablespoons finely chopped vegetable cubes (leek, celery root (celeriac), carrots or carrots and peas)
1½ dl vegetable broth
Kelpamare
rosemary
1 tablespoon olive oil and 10 g nut spread

Sauté onion, diced vegetable and hot-rinsed millet until glazed. Add hot vegetable broth, season and boil for 20 min. Before serving, top with olive oil or butter.

Coarse-ground grain mash
2 tablespoons coarse-ground grain (wheat, oats, rye)
3 tablespoons water
1 pinch rock salt

Soak the coarse-ground grain for 12 hours then boil in water for 10 min. or cook for ½ hour in a bain-marie.

Pasta, spaghetti, macaroni, etc.
For a strict healing diet, egg pasta should not be used. Today there also are high quality wholegrain pastas, soy pastas and spelt pastas in addition to the well-known Italian pasta products made from wheat. Note that there are many sauces which we cannot recommend.

The best-tolerated pasta products are cooked al dente with a classic or simple tomato sauce (see recipes page 125).

Spätzle or Knöpfli (without egg)
60 g wholegrain flour
20 g soy flour
1 dl 1:1 diluted milk
1 l water
1 tablespoon rock salt
1 tablespoon olive oil

onion, julienned
chives and parsley

Mix wholegrain and soy flour thoroughly with diluted milk and tap the mixture until the dough forms bubbles. Let rest for at least 1 hour. Boil water with rock salt. Press the dough in portions through a coarse screen into the boiling water or put it onto a small wooden cutting board. Cut fine strips with a knife and place them in the boiling water. Let the Knöpfli or Spätzle simmer until they rise to the surface. Take them out with a skimmer and place them on a hot platter. As desired, garnish with julienned onion sautéed in olive oil (or without fat), chives and parsley.

Sauces

Sauces are a challenge for those on a healing diet, since almost all sauce recipes contain fat (butter, oil, cream), cheese and eggs. The combination of hot fat and flour (béchamel sauce) should always be avoided, because this mixture is very hard on the stomach, liver and intestines. We have put together a few adapted sauces here, whose recipes deviate from the classical ones. All of them taste great!

Béchamel sauce 1
For 4 persons

2–3 tablespoons wheat flour (white flour may be used exceptionally)
1 l milk
1 bay leaf
1 tablespoon vegetable broth
1 grated onion
1 pinch each rock salt, nutmeg and freshly ground white pepper
chopped parsley

Briefly cook the flour in a sauce pan until it is aromatic (it must not turn dark), then let it cool slightly. Add the milk while stirring constantly. Add the bay leaf, vegetable broth and onion and bring to a boil. Season. After approx. 5 minutes, remove the bay leaf and serve the sauce sprinkled with parsley.

This basic sauce can be used to make many versions. For example:

Horseradish sauce
At the end, add 10 g finely grated horseradish and cook the sauce for another 5 min.

Caper sauce
Season the finished sauce with whole or chopped capers and lemon juice.

Olive sauce
Briefly cook the sauce with 4–5 tablespoons tomato pulp and 2 tablespoons chopped olives. Season with a knife point of cayenne pepper (optional).

Herb sauce
Mix plenty of finely chopped herbs such as parsley, lovage, chervil, basil, estragon, oregano, etc. into the finished sauce.

Champignon sauce
Mix 3–4 tablespoons of very finely chopped raw champignons into the finished sauce and season with lemon juice.

Béchamel sauce 2
For 4 persons

2 tablespoons wheat flour
½ l soy milk
1 bay leaf
1 onion, finely grated
2 teaspoons red miso
1 pinch each of pepper and paprika
chopped parsley

Briefly brown the flour without fat until it gives off a toasted aroma. Let it cool a little, then add the soy milk while stirring constantly. Add the bay leaf and onion and boil for about 5 min.

Stir in the miso, remove the bay leaf and season the sauce with pepper and paprika. Sprinkle with chopped parsley.

Miso is a fermented soy bean paste that is great for seasoning. It tastes like soy sauce but does not contain salt.

Tomato sauce, classic
½ tablespoon olive oil
1 tablespoon onion
½ garlic clove, pressed
2 tablespoons carrot, celery, leek
2 small tomatoes
1 pinch rock salt
1 pinch raw cane sugar
1 teaspoon tomato puree
1½ dl vegetable broth or water
bay leaf, rosemary, thyme

Sauté the chopped onion, pressed garlic and coarsely cut vegetables in olive oil. Add the diced tomatoes and the tomato puree, then add vegetable broth (or water). Season and simmer for ½ hour. Strain if desired.

Tomato sauce, simple
3 tomatoes
1 pinch each rock salt and raw cane sugar (Sucanat)
chives, basil
1 tablespoon olive oil
Dice tomatoes, cook over low heat, season and strain. Add olive oil to taste.

Sweet pepper sauce
½ tablespoon olive oil
1 tablespoon onion, chopped
1 tablespoon sweet pepper (yellow, green or red)
1 tablespoon wholemeal flour
1 dl vegetable broth
1 pinch rock salt
1 tablespoon cream (optional)

Lightly sauté onions and finely sliced sweet pepper in olive oil. Sprinkle with wholegrain flour, add vegetable broth and cook for 20 min. Season. Fold cream into the finished sauce to enrich.

Mayonnaise, classic
For 4 persons

1 egg yolk
1 tablespoon lemon juice
2 dl olive oil
onion, herbs, Kelpamare

Mix the egg yolk well with several drops of lemon juice. Add the oil drop by drop while stirring evenly with the whisk. If the mayonnaise grows too thick, dilute with lemon juice. Season to taste.

Remoulade sauce, classic
For 4 persons

Prepare mayonnaise according to above recipe
1 hard-boiled egg, chopped
1 tablespoon cornichons, chopped
some capers
1 teaspoon parsley, chopped
small tomato diced

Mix the various ingredients with the finished mayonnaise. Garnish with diced tomato.

Mayonnaise without animal protein
See recipe page 106

Remoulade sauce without animal protein
For 4 persons
Prepare mayonnaise without animal protein (see recipe page 106) and mix with 1 tablespoon chopped cornichons, capers and chopped parsley. Garnish with diced tomato.

Vinaigrette
For 4 persons

2 tablespoons olive oil
2 tablespoons groundnut oil
2½ tablespoons lemon juice
2 tablespoons water or vegetable broth

½ onion, chopped
1 egg, hard boiled and chopped
1–2 cornichons, cut or finely chopped
parsley or chives
1 tablespoon small tomato, diced
1 pinch rock salt

Whisk olive oil, lemon juice and vegetable broth until smooth, then add the other ingredients, mixing thoroughly.

Sandwiches

Sandwiches are generally popular as appetizers, for a summer meal, to take along on hikes and trips, and as lunch at the office. Spreads and ingredients can be used in any number of ways, and various wholegrain bread types are available, some pre-sliced.

The recipes are for 4 persons.

Basic spreads
For the strict diet, spread some quark on the bread rolls and add raw food.

Guacamole (South American avocado mousse)
2 ripe avocados
juice of ½ lemon
½ small onion, chopped
2 garlic cloves, pressed
rock salt and white pepper (optional)

Mash the flesh removed from the avocados with the lemon juice in a blender. Mix in onion and garlic and season with rock salt and white pepper. If desired, stir in 1 tablespoon soy cream (instead of crème fraiche).

Sweet avocado cream
1 ripe avocado
4 tablespoons fresh orange juice
1 tablespoon honey
1 knife tip ginger powder

Mash the pulp removed from the avocado by squeezing or blending it and mix in the other ingredients. Serve at once.

Tofu spread with nuts
250 g tofu, pureed
2 finely chopped spring onions
50 g nuts (hazelnuts, walnuts, almonds, cashews)
1 pinch rock salt and white pepper (optional)

Lightly roast the nuts in the oven or a dry pan, let them cool and then grind them up. Mix with the pureed tofu and onion. Season with rock salt and pepper.

Quark spread with herbs
100 g quark
10 g nut spread
miso
caraway, chives or herbs (dill, borage, lovage, basil, oregano, peppermint etc.)

Stir quark and nut spread to a frothy consistency, season and add individual herbs (or a mix) for variety.

Garnishes
Spreads can be garnished in the following ways:
with raw carrots or celery
with tomatoes, fresh cucumbers, radish, cress, onion, nuts, parsley, chives etc.

Desserts

These recipes are for 4 persons.

Desserts should be eaten with great restraint. Use honey (acacia honey is particularly good), maple syrup or agave juice to sweeten. Do not eat any sweet dishes with large quantities of sugar, eggs or cream. There are many tasty alternatives!

Fruit salad
2 tablespoons honey
1 dl water
1–2 dl grape juice or apple juice
1–2 tablespoons lemon juice
600 g apricots or peaches (seasonal)
melons
apples
pears (ripe)
red cherries, pitted
berries

Mix thoroughly water, honey, grape juice and lemon juice. Thinly slice fruits and add them to the syrup.

Filled melons
2 small melons
fruit salad as per recipe above

Halve the melons, scoop out the seeds and fill the melons with the fruit salad.

Fruit jelly
3 dl water or grape juice
1–2 tablespoons honey
10 g agar-agar, powdered
7 dl fresh orange or berry juice

Agar-agar is a plant-based gelatine powder that is used for vegetable and fruit spreads, sauces and puddings, etc. instead of animal gelatine.

Mix water, honey and agar-agar and cook over low heat while stirring constantly until the agar-agar has dissolved. Add fruit juice and serve immediately in glasses or desert cups. Garnish with sesame cream (see recipe page 109).

Apple sauce
800 g apples
2 dl water or apple juice
1–2 tablespoons honey
cinnamon or lemon peel (from untreated lemon)
1 dl sesame cream (see recipe page 109)

Core and cut the apples into pieces, cook them in the water or apple juice and honey until soft, and strain them. Mix with cinnamon or lemon peel (from untreated lemons). To enrich, serve sesame cream with the apple sauce.

Apple or pear compote
800 g apples or pears
2–3 dl water or apple juice
1 tablespoon honey
grated lemon peel (from untreated lemons) or a little cinnamon

Core and peel the apples or pears, and cut them into wedges. Bring water or juice to a boil, add honey and lemon peel or cinnamon, add the fruit, and cook until soft.

Baked apples (recipe 1)
800 g apples
½ l water or apple juice
1 tablespoon honey
¼ cinnamon stick
quince, raspberry or currant jelly (see recipe page 127)
or raisins and wine berries with a little honey

Boil water or apple juice with honey and cinnamon stick. Peel, core, halve and place apples in portions in the hot water or juice. Cook slowly until soft. Remove with skimmer and place on a flat platter with the cut surface up. Fill the apples with jelly or mix of raisin, wine, berry and honey.

Baked apples (recipe 2)
4 large or 8 small apples
4 tablespoons ground hazelnuts or almonds
2 tablespoons currants
4 tablespoons sesame cream (see recipe page 109)
1–2 tablespoons honey
grated lemon peel (untreated lemon)

10 g nut spread
1 tablespoon maple syrup
1–2 dl apple juice

Mix hazelnuts, currants, sesame cream, honey and lemon peel, fill the prepared apples (cored and peeled) and place the apples in a casserole. Add nut spread and maple syrup and pour 1 cm. apple juice over the apples. Bake for 20–30 min.

Dried fruit salad with grapes and pine nuts
200 g dried figs
200 g dates
200 g dried apples
400 g white grapes
juice of 1 lemon
2 tablespoons honey
50 g pine nuts

Chop the dried fruit, halve one-half of the grapes and squeeze the others. Put all fruits in a dish. Mix the lemon and grape juice with the honey and pour it over the fruit. Cool before serving. Toast the pine nuts and sprinkle them over the fruit salad.

Strawberry or raspberry cream
300 g berries
vanilla cream
1–2 dl sesame cream (see recipe page 109)

Prepare a vanilla cream according to the recipe on page 129 and mix with the mixed or pureed berries. Fold in sesame cream or serve separately.

Lemon cream
¾ l milk
1–2 lemons, untreated
1 tablespoon cornflour or arrowroot flour
3 tablespoons milk
2 tablespoons honey
sesame cream (see recipe page 109) to taste

Thinly slice the lemon peel and boil in the milk. Add cornflour or arrowroot flour stirred with a little cold milk and the honey and boil briefly. Add honey and return to the pan, stirring constantly, and heat almost to the boil. Strain the cooled cream, and add a few spoons of lemon juice and sesame cream to taste.

Orange cream
Prepare as lemon cream (see recipe above)

Orange aspics
5 dl orange juice
5 g agar-agar, powdered (plant jelly instead of gelatine)
1 tablespoon fruit sugar

Mix 3 dl orange juice, agar-agar and sugar and heat over a low flame while stirring constantly (do not boil) until the agar-agar has dissolved completely. Add the remaining orange juice and pour it into chilled moulds. Let cool.

Sesame bars
100 g Syramena sugar
2 tablespoons honey
100 g sesame seeds, not ground

Syramena sugar is a light raw-cane sugar available in organic food stores. Heat the sugar in a dry pan and stir until a light caramel forms. Add the liquid honey and mix well. Add the sesame and mix well again. Pour the mass into a mould or onto an oiled board, let cool slightly and cut into squares or diamonds. Let cool.

Vanilla cream
1 vanilla pod
¼ l water
40 g wheat flour (white flour may be used exceptionally)
3 tablespoons honey
approx. 200 ml soy milk

Split the vanilla pod lengthwise, scrape the seeds into the water, add the pod and bring to the boil. Put the wheat flour into the vanilla water while stirring constantly and let it swell into a thick mash. Let it cool a little, then stir in the honey and soy milk. Depending on the amount of soy milk, you will get vanilla cream or vanilla sauce. Keep cool until serving.

Vanilla sauce
See vanilla cream (recipe above)

Almond-milk sauce
4 dl milk
50 g almonds or almond spread
2 tablespoons honey
1 tablespoon cornflour or arrowroot flour
2 tablespoons water

Boil milk with the peeled, ground almonds (or the almond spread) and honey. Stir cornflour or arrowroot flour in cold water and stir into the boiling milk. Mix the finished sauce.

Rosehip sauce
70 g rosehip puree or rosehip pulp
2 dl water or grape juice
1–2 tablespoons honey
a few drops of lemon juice (optional)

Boil the ingredients together, then add the lemon juice.

Red-wine sauce
2 dl water
lemon or orange peel (untreated fruits)
1 cinnamon stalk
1 clove
1–2 tablespoons honey
2 dl red grape juice
20 g almonds

Boil water, peel, spices and honey together for a few min., then strain. Add grape juice and heat (do not boil). Add peeled and sliced almonds.

Red fruit jelly (iced soup)
7 dl currant, raspberry or strawberry juice
3 dl red grape juice or water
70 g semolina
1 tablespoon cornflour

Boil berry juice and grape juice together, stir in semolina and cornflour and boil for 10 min. Pour into rinsed pudding mould and cool.
Serve with vanilla sauce (see recipe page 129) or almond-milk sauce (see recipe page 129).

Red fruit jelly, Danish style
1 kg berries (raspberries, currants, strawberries or pitted cherries, or a mix)
1 l fruit juice (e.g. elderberry)
2 packs of agar-agar
honey to taste
½ teaspoon natural vanilla
sesame cream, liquid (see recipe page 109)

Put cleaned and chopped (optional) fruits into a dish, mix with honey and vanilla. Heat the fruit juice with agar-agar and pour the liquid over the fruits. Let the fruit jelly harden. Serve with liquid sesame cream.

Table for Raw Food Diet

Preparation	Treatment	Effect	Duration	Quantity
juice: fruit, raw vegetables plant milk (almond soy, sesame) certified raw milk, if prescribed, additions of whole cereal or flax seed gruel (always ⅓ of the juice) or cream and a little lemon juice	General metabolism overload (fasting indication), obesity, heart and circulatory failure, gastro-intestinal, kidney and liver inflammations, acute flu (fever)	Detoxifying, relieving, dewatering (relieves heart and circulation), seals vessels, reduces inflammation, de-acidifying, promotes nutritional economy, restores the intestinal milieu, reduces weight	1–28 days depending on medical prescription; 1–3 days for longer fasting treatments	600–800 g fresh juices (3–4 glasses) 450–500 g plant milk or herbal tea, 200–400 calories
Pureed (slightly greater quantity, oil added): fruit and vegetables mixed in the blender (vegetables with sauce, see recipes), plant milk (almond, soy, sesame), certified raw milk, sour milk, butter milk, whey, yoghurt	Inflammations in the digestive system, convalescence	Same as juice, plus cellulose content (stimulation of the peristalsis), addition of oil	3–14 days depending on medical prescription	Approx. 1200 calories (see daily menu)

Healthful teas

Use whole leaves for teas if possible, since essential oils are lost when the leaves are chopped finely (sachet form). Bitter and flatulence teas should be drunk unsweetened, while other teas may be enhanced with honey and/or lemon juice

Bitter tea
Wormwood
Centaurium
Cnicus

Mix in equal parts, boil briefly and steep for 5 min.
To stimulate the appetite, drink 2–3 tablespoons ½ hour before meals (mildly cholagogic).
Sensitive persons should use only centaurium.

Wormwood tea
Boil slightly and steep for 5 min.
Strong bitter tea, strongly cholagogic, stimulates gastric juices.
Drink in sips throughout the day.

Flatulence tea
Caraway
Fennel
Aniseed

Mix in equal parts, boil briefly and steep for 20 min.
Drink 1 cup after meals to prevent flatulence.

Chamomile tea
Boil briefly and steep. (Otherwise risk of nausea, even vomiting)

For stomach pain.
Cleansing and calming effect on the gastrointestinal tract.
For enemas and rinsing.

Peppermint tea
Boil briefly.
Calming, cholagogic.

Vervain tea
Boil briefly.
Calming, mucous reducing, cholagogic; very popular in France.

Lemon balm tea
Boil briefly.
Very calming, good before bedtime.

Lemon peel tea
Thinly cut off the peel of 1 untreated lemon, boil for approx. 5 min. with ½ l water, let steep for 10 min. and strain.

Orange blossom tea
Boil 2–3 blossoms for 2–3 min., let steep and strain. Sweeten with honey.
Calming; drink at bedtime.

Flax seed tea
Boil 1 tablespoon linseeds in ½ l water for 7–10 min. and let steep.
Mucous reducing, mildly laxative.

Lady's mantle tea
Briefly boil 2 tablespoons of leaves in ½ l water, steep for 10 min.
Prevents gynaecological problems.

Alpine lady's mantle tea
Like lady's-mantle tea.

Solidago tea
(golden rod, baneberry)

Boil 1 tablespoon solidago in ½ l water for 1 min., let simmer for 10 min.
For dropsy, bladder and kidney infections; water expelling.
2–3 cups per day.

Water expelling (diuretic), stimulates the creation of primary urine in the kidneys.

Bearberry leaf tea
Briefly boil 1½ tablespoons bearberry leaves in 5 dl water for 5 min., steep for 10 min. and strain.
For bladder infections.

Lavender tea
Briefly boil 1 teaspoon lavender leaves, steep briefly.
Calming, harmonising, anti-inflammatory; for sleeplessness.

Rosehip tea
Soak 2–3 tablespoons rosehip seeds and peels in 1½ l water for 12 hours, boil gently for ½–¾ hours and strain. The next day the boiled rosehips can be boiled again with fresh ones.
Slightly cholagogic and water expelling (diuretic).

Recipes

Almond milk	109
Almond milk of fresh almonds	109
Almond milk sauce	129
Almond or sesame puree dressing	106
Alpine lady's mantle tea	131
Apple or pear compote	128
Apple sauce	127
Artichokes	117
Asparagus	117
Ayurveda potatoes	121
Baked apples (recipe 1)	128
Baked apples (recipe 2)	128
Baked fennel with cream cheese	114
Baked potatoes	120
Basic spreads	126
Bearberry leaf tea	132
Béchamel sauce 1	124
Béchamel sauce 2	125
Bircher muesli	101
Bircher muesli with almond or sesame puree	101
Bircher muesli with berries or stone fruit	102
Bircher muesli with condensed milk	103
Bircher muesli with dried fruits	102
Bircher muesli with orange juice	102
Bircher muesli with various fruits	102
Bircher muesli with yoghurt, sour or buttermilk	102
Bitter tea	131
Bouillon potatoes	120
Butter, fresh	109
Caper sauce	125
Caraway potatoes	120
Carrots, cooked	115
Cauliflower or broccoli	118
Celery root (celeriac) salad with soy mayonnaise	119
Celery root (celeriac), steamed	115
Celery stalks	114
Celery with béchamel sauce	116
Chamomile tea	131
Champignon sauce	125
Chard with béchamel sauce	114
Chervil soup	113
Coarse-ground grain mash	124
Cold-pressed sunflower oil, corn seed oil, thistle oil, cold-pressed olive oil	110
Corn on the cob	118
Courgettes with tomatoes	117
Cream dressing	105
Creamed potatoes	120
Dried fruit salad with grapes and pine seeds	128
Endive/chicory	114
Filled melons	127
Flatulence tea	131
Flax seed Gruel	101
Flax seed tea	131
Fruit jelly	127
Fruit salad	127
Garlic dressing	106
Garnishes	127
Green beans with tomatoes	115
Guacamole (South American avocado mousse)	126

Health-food store vegetable margarine and health-food store food fats	109
Herbal soup	111
Herb sauce	125
Horseradish sauce	125
Indian rice dish	123
Japanese rice	122
Jerusalem artichoke	116
Kohlrabi with herbs	118
Lady's mantle tea	131
Lavender tea	132
Lemon balm tea	131
Lemon crème	128
Lemon dressing	105
Lemon peel tea	131
Lettuce	114
Linomel muesli according to Dr. Johanna Budwig	103
Mayonnaise, classic	126
Mayonnaise without animal protein	126
Mayonnaise with wholegrain soy flour instead of egg	106
Millet risotto	123
Millet risotto with vegetables	124
Minestrone	113
Nut dressing	106
Nut spread and almond puree	110
Oat cream soup	111
Oat groat soup	112
Oil dressing	105
Olive oil	109
Olive sauce	125
Orange aspics	129
Orange blossom tea	131
Orange cream	129
Orange dressing	105
Pasta, spaghetti, macaroni, etc.	124
Peas and carrots	115

Peas, French style	115
Peppermint dressing	106
Peppermint tea	131
Pine nut milk	109
Polenta	123
Potatoes in their skins	119
Potatoes, mashed	120
Potatoes with tomatoes	120
Potato goulash	121
Potato puree	121
Potato salad	118
Potato salad with cucumbers	118
Potato slices with spinach	121
Potato soup	113
Quark dressing	105
Quark potatoes	120
Quark spread with herbs	127
Ratatouille	117
Red beets	116
Red fruit jelly, Danish style	130
Red fruit jelly (iced soup)	130
Red wine sauce	129
Remoulade sauce, classic	126
Remoulade sauce without animal protein	126
Rice gratin with tomatoes	123
Rice or barley gruel	101
Rice salad	119
Rice soup, clear	111
Rice soup, thickened	111
Rice with courgettes	122
Rice with spinach	122
Risi bisi (rice with peas)	122
Risotto	122
Riz creole with vegetables	122
Roast potatoes	121
Rosehip sauce	129
Rosehip tea	132
Saffron rice	122
Salade niçoise	119
Sauerkraut salad	107
Sautéed chicory	114
Semolina mash	123
Semolina soup	112
Sesame bars	129
Sesame cream	109

Sesame frappé	109	Tomatoes, stewed	116
Sesame milk	109	Tomatoes, stuffed	116
Solidago tea	131	Tomato rice	122
Soy milk	109	Tomato sauce, classic	125
Spätzle or Knöpfli (without egg)	124	Tomato sauce, simple	125
Spinach, chopped	113	Tomato soup	112
Spinach, whole leaves (and stems)	114	Tomato soup, summer	112
Sprouted cereal grains	103	Vanilla cream	129
Strawberry or raspberry cream	128	Vegetable aspics	119
		Vegetable bouillon	111
		Vegetable broth	111
Sugar peas (snow peas), cooked	115	Vegetable curry	115
Sweet avocado cream	126	Vegetable soups (carrots, spinach, broccoli)	112
Sweet pepper sauce	125	Vervain tea	131
Sweet peppers, green, yellow, red	117	Vinaigrette	126
		Wormwood tea	131
Tofu spread with nuts	127		
Tomatoes à la provençale	117	Yoghurt dressing	105
Tomatoes, steamed	116		

Notes

1 American Heart Association, Inc., 'Cardiovascular disease, statistics 2006', Interneteintrag 2010.
2 Joseph, A. et al., 'Manifestations of coronary artherosclerosis in young trauma victims – an autopsy study', *J. Am. Coll. Cardiol.* 1993 Aug 22 (2459–67).
3 Massin, M.M. et al., 'Arteriosclerosis lifestyle risk factors in children with congenital heart disease', *Eur J Cardiocasc Prev Rehabil* 2007 Apr: 14(2): 349–51.
4 Gerber, Z.R. et al., 'Risk factors for atherosclerosis in children: an epidemiologic study', *Arg Bras Cardiol* 1997 Oct, 69(4): 231–6.
5 Gupta, R. et al., 'Prevalence of atherosclerosis risk factors in adolescent school children', *Indian Heart J.* 1998 Sep-Oct, 50(5): 511–5.
6 Strong, J.P. et al., 'Early lesions of atherosclerosis in childhood and youth: natural history and risk factors', *J Am Coll Nutr* 1992 Jun 11; Suppl 51S–54S.
7 Tanaka, K. et al., 'A nationwide study of atherosclerosis in infants, children and young adults in Japan', *Atherosclerosis* 1988 Aug 72(2–3): 143–56.
8 Hochrein, M., in *Ärzte sprechen zu dir.* Med. Verlag Hans Huber, Bern, 1956.
9 Eppinger, H., *Einiges über diätetische Therapie* Zeitschrift für ärztliche Fortbildung, Verlag Gustav Fischer, Jena, 36.Jg. Nr. 22 u 23, 673–678, 709–714,1939.
10 Pischinger, A. et al., *Das System der Grundregulation. Grundlagen für eine ganzheits-biologische Theorie der Medizin* (1990). 8. Auflage, Haug-Verlag, Heidelberg.
11 Bischof, M., *Biophotonen, das Licht in unseren Zellen,* ISBN 3–86150-095-7.
12 Popp, F.A., *Biologie des Lichtes, Grundlagen der ultraschwachen Zellstrahlung,* Verlag Paul Parey ISBN 3-489-61734-7.
13 Rubik, B., *Natural light from organisms Life at the edge of science,* p. 123, and Fischer, H., *Photons as transmitter for intra- and intercellular biological and biochemical communication – the construction of a hypothesis. Electromagnetic bio-information,* F.A. Popp, ed., Urban & Schwarzenberg, Munich, 1989, p.70.
14 Van Vijck, R. and E., Utrecht Univerity, *An introduction to Human Biophoton Emission,* Forsch Komplementärmed Klass Naturheilkd. 1005, 12 S. 77–83.
15 Bircher-Benner, M.O., *Grundzüge der Ernährungstherapie auf Grund der Energie-Spannung der Nahrung,* Verlag Otto Salle, Berlin, 1905 and 1906.
16 Bircher-Benner, M.O., *Der zweite Hauptsatz der Energetik und die Ernährung.* Zeitschr der Wendepunkt, Wendepunkt-Verlag, Zürich, 1936.
17 Bircher-Benner, M.O., *Vom Wesen und der Organisation der Nahrungsenergie und über die Anwendung des zweiten Hauptsatzes der Energielehre auf den Nährwert und die Nahrungswirkung.* Kleine Hippokratesbücherei Band 8, Hippokrates-Verlag Stuttgart and Leipzig.
18 Popp, F.A., *Unsere Lebensmittel in neuer Sicht,* ISBN 3-596-11457-4.
19 Stary, H.C., 'Evolution and progression of atherosclerosis lesions in coronary arteries of children and young adults, arteriosclerosis', journal article, university research support, U.S. Gov't P.H.S. Louisiana State University, School of Medicine, New Orleans, 70112.
20 Gerber, Z.R. et al., 'Risk factors for coronary arteriosclerosis in children: an epidemiologic study', *Arg Bras Cardiol,* 1997 Oct; 69(4): 231–6, MEDLINE PMID 9595714.
21 Gupta, R. et al., 'Prevalence of atherosclerosis risk factors in adolescent school children', *Indian Heart J.* 1998 Sep–Oct; 50(5): *Indian Heart J* 1994 May–Jun, vol 56(3) 146–9, ISSN 0019-4832.511–5.
22 Strong, J.P. et al., 'Early lesions of atherosclerosis in childhood and youth: natural history and risk factors', *J Am Col Nutr.* 1992 Jun 11 Suppl 51S S. 545.
23 Tanaka, K. et al., 'A nation-wide study of atherosclerosis in infants, children and young adults in Japan', *Atherosclerosis* 1988 Aug. 72(2–3), 143–56.
24 Joseph, A. et al., 'Manifestations of coronary ath-

erosclerosis in young trauma victims: an autopsy study', *J. Am. Coll. Cardiol.* 1993 Aug: 22(2): 459–67.
25. Steinberger, J. et al., 'AHA Scientific Statement: Obesity, Insulin Resistance, Diabetes, and Cardiovascular Risk in Children', *Circ. AHA journals*, org 2003: 107: 1448–53.
26. Wilbert-Lampen, U. et al., 'Cardiovsacular Events during World Cup Soccer', *New Engl J. of Med.* 358, Nr. 5, 2008, 475–483.
27. Powel, L. H., 'Emotional Arousal as a Predictor of Long-Term Mortality and Morbidity in Post M. l. Men', *Circulation*, Band 82, 4, Supplem III, October 1990.
28. Mittleman, M.A. et al., 'Triggering of acute myocardial infarction onset by episodes of anger: Determinants of Myocardial Infarction Onset Study Investigators', *Circulation* 92 Nr 7 Oct 1995 1720–25.
29. Rme/aerzteblatt.de: *Migräne mit Aura als Herzinfarkt- und Thromboserisiko* (http///www.aerzteblatt.de/nachrichten/53048/. Abgerufen am 26.12.2014.
30. Hill/aerzteblatt.de: *mehr Herzinfarkte in ärmeren Stadtteilen* Aerzteblatt.de. 4. September 2013, abgerufen am 26. Dezember 2014.
31. Statistisches Bundesamt *Tabellen*, abgerufen am 17.1.2013, https//www.statistis.de.
32. Gupta, R. et al., 'Influence of alcohol intake on high density lipoprotein cholesterol levels in middle-aged men'.
33. Tsuare, S. et al., 'Alcohol consumption and all-cause and cancer mortality among middle-aged Japanese men: seven year follow up of the JPIIC-Study rohort I', Japan Public Health Center. *Am. J. of epidemiology*, 1999, Dec a Vol 150(11) p.1201–07. ISSN 0002–9262.
34. Gisling, E., *Check-up Nr. 6* 1994, S. 4 Infomed-Verlag, CH9500 Wil.
35. Whitby, G.F. et al., 'Developmental effects of combined exposure to ethanol and vitamin A', *Food-ChemF-toxical* 1994 Apr. vol. 32(4), 305–20, ISSN 0278–6915.
36. Waagh, M. et al., 'Effect of social drinking on neuropsychological performance', *Br-J-Addict* 1989 Jun, vol: 84(6), P: 659–67, ISSN: 0952–0482.
37. Parker, E.S. et al., 'Alcohol and the disruption of cognitive processes', *Arch. Gen Psychiary* 1974 Dec vol 31 (6) 824–8. ISSN: 0003–990X.
38. Voytechowsky, M. et al., 'The influence of alcohol on memory functions in healthy volunteers', *Act-Nerv-Saper* (Praha) 1970, vol 12(3), 255–6.
39. Wannametzee, G. et al., 'Alcohol and sudden cardiac death', a paper of the Department of Public Health and Primary Care, Royal Free Hospital School of Medicine, London, NW 32 PF, 1992.
40. EPIC-Symosium, Berlin: *Was schützt vor Krebs und Diabetes? Konsensuserklärung* MMW-Fortschr. Med. Nr. 24/2007 (149 jg) S. 16, 25.4.2007.
41. Harman, D., 'Aging: a theory based on free radical and radiation chemistry', *J of Gerontology* 11, 1956 S. 298–300 PMID 13332224.
42. Harman, D., 'The free radical theory of aging', *Antioxid Redox Signal* 5, 2003, S. 557–561, PMID 14580310.
43. Bockman, K.B. et al., 'Mitochondrial aging: open questions', *Ann N.Y. Acad Sci* 854, 1998, S. 118–127, PMID 9928425.
44. Sohr, Ch., 'Oxidativer Stress bei diabetischer Neuropahtie', Medizinische Fakultiät, Deutsches Diabetes-Zentrum DDZ, 2007 (online).
45. Eppinger, H., *Die Permeabilitätspathologie als die Lehre vom Krankheitsbeginn,* Springer-Verlag Wien, 1949.
46. Bircher-Benner, M.O., *Vegetabile Heilkost,* Klinische Fortbildung in Neue deutsche Klinik, Ergänzungsband, 110–168, 1937.
47. Astrup, A. et al., 'Dietary fibre added to very low calorie reduced hunger and alleviates constipation', *J-Obes* 1990 Feb, vol: 14(2), 109–12, ISSN 0307–6565.
48. Barlow, C.W. et al., 'Effects of therapy with diet and simvastatin on atherosclerosis in hypercholesterolemic patients', *Cardiovasc-Drugs-Ther.,* 1990 Oct, vol: 4(5) 1389–94, ISSN 0920–3206.
49. White, J.L. et al., 'Oat bran lowers plasma cholesterol levels in mildly hypercholesterolemic men', *J Am Diet Assoc* 1992 Apr vol 92(4) 446–9 m USSB; 0002–8223.
50. Bae, C.Y. et al., 'Clinical Trial of American Heart Association step one diet for treatment of hypercholesterolemics', *J Cam Pract* 1991 Sept, vol: 33(3) 249–54, ISSN: 0094–3509.
51. Keenan, J.M. et al., 'Randomised, controlled, crossover trial of oat bran in hypercholesterolemic subjects', *J Fam Pract* 1991 Dec, vol 33(6), P 6608, ISSN 0094–3509.
52. Cara, L. et al., 'Plasma lipid lowering effects of

52. wheat germ in hypercholesterolemic subjects', *Plant Foods Hum Nutr* 1991 Apr, vol: 41(2) 135–50, ISSN 0921–9668.
53. Bell, L.P. et al., 'Cholesterol-lowering effects of soluble fibre cereals as part of a prudent diet for patients with mild to moderate hypercholesterolemia', *Am J Clin Nutr.* 1990 Dec, vol: 52(6) 1020–26, ISSN 002–9165.
54. Neal, G.W. et al., 'Synergetic effects of Psyllium in dietary treatment of hypercholesterolemia', *South Med J* 1990 Oct col: 83(10) 1131–37, ISSN 0038–4348.
55. Levin, E.G. et al., 'Compensation of psyllium hydrophilic mucilloid and celllulose as adjuncts to prudent diet in the treatment of mild to moderate hypercholesterolemia', *Arch Int Med* 1990 sep vol 150(9) 1822–27, ISSN 003–9926.
56. Skuladottir, G.V. et al., 'Influence of dietary cod liver oil on fatty acid composition of plasma lipids in human male subjects after myocardial infarction', *J intern Med* 1990 Dec vol 228(6) 563–68. ISSN 0954–6820.
57. Gans, R.O. et al., 'Fish-oil supplementation in patients with stable claudication', *Am J Surg* 1990 Nov vol 160(5) 490–95, ISSN 0002–9610.
58. D'Amico, G. et al., 'Effect of dietary proteins and lipids in patients with membranous nephropathy and nephrotic syndrome', *Clin Nephrol* 1991 Jun vol 36(6) 237–42, ISSN 0301–0430.
59. Singh, R.B. et al., 'Randomised controlled trial of cardio-protective diet in patients with recent acute myocardial infarction: results of one year follow up' *BMJ* 1992 Apr 18 vol 304(6833) 1015–19, ISSN 0959–8138.
60. Yinnon, A.M. et al., 'A practical level in primary care', *Fam Prat* 1992 Jan vol 9(2) 167–70, ISSN 0028–4793.
61. Sciarrone, S.E. et al., 'A factorial study of salt restriction and a low-fat/high fibre diet in hypertensive subjects', *J Hapertens* 1992 Mar vol 10(3) 287–98, ISSN 0263–6352.
62. Melchert, H.U., 'Fatty acid pattern in triglycerides, diglycerides, free fatty acids, cholesteryl ester and phosphatidylcholine in serum from vegetarians', *Atherosclerosis* 1987 May vol 65(1–2) 159–66, ISSN 0021–9150.
63. Gotto, A.M. et al., 'Rationale for treatment', *Am J Med* 1991 Jul 31 vol 91 (1B) 315–365, ISSN 002–9343 18.
64. Wood, P.D. et al., 'The effects on Plasma Lipoproteins of a prudent weight-reducing diet, with or without exercise in overweight men and women', *New Engl J Med* 1991 A4g 15 vol 325(7) 461–6. ISSN 0028–4793.
65. Ornish, D. et al., 'Can Lifestyle changes reverse coronary heart disease? The Lifestyle Heart Trial' (see comments), *Lancet* 1990 Jul 21, vol 336(8708) 129–33, ISSN 0023–7507.
66. Dougall, J. et al., 'Rapid reduction of serum cholesterol and blood pressure by a twelve day, very low fat, strictly vegetarian diet', *J Am Coll Nutr* 1995 Dec 1 vol. 14(5) 491–96 ISSN 0731–5724.
67. Chang, C.J. et al., 'Mortality pattern of German vegetarians after 11 years of follow-up' (see comments), *Epidemiology* 1992 Sep vol 3(5) 395–401, ISSN 1044–3983.
68. Ritter, M.M. et al., 'Effects of vegetarian lifestyle on health', *Fortschritt Med* 1995 Jun 10 vol 114(16) 239–42, ISSN 0015–8178.
69. Chang, C.J. et al., 'Dietary and Lifestyle determinants of mortality among German vegetarians', Division of Epidemiology, Germen Cancer Research Center, Heidelberg, *Int J Epidemiol* 1993 Apr vol 22(2) 228–36, ISSN 0300–5771.
70. Rottka, H., 'Health and vegetarian lifestyle', *Bibl. Nutr. Pieta* 1990(45) 176–94, ISSN 0067–8198-66 Refs.
71. Rich, H. G., 'Resolution of focal fatty infiltration of the liver', *South Med J* 1996 Oct vol 89(10) 1024–27 Refs, ISSN 0038–4348.
72. Park, H.S. et al., 'Effects of weight control on hepatic abnormalities in obese patients with fatty liver', *J Korean Med* S 1995 Dec vol 10(6) 414–21, ISSN 1011–8934.
73. Ueno, T. et al., 'Therapeutic effects of restricted diet and exercise in obese patients with fatty liver', *J Hepatol* 1997 Jul vol 27(1) 103–7, ISSN 0168–8278.
74. Heshka, S. et al., 'Obesity and risk of gall stone development on a 1200 Kcal regular food diet' (see comments), *Int J Obes Relat Metab Disord* 1996 May vol 20/5) 430–34, ISBN 0307–0565.
75. Christl, S. U. et al., 'Fatty liver in adult celiac disease', *Deutsche Med Wochenschr* 1999 June 4, vol 124(22) 691–94, ISSN 0012–1472.
76. Schwinghackl, L. et al., 'Effects of Monounsaturated Fatty Acids on glycaemic control in patients with abnormal glucose metabolism: a systemic

review and meta-analysis', *Ann Nutr Metab* 2011; 58290–96, doi.10.1159/000331214.

77 Schwinghackl, L. et al., 'Effect of monounsaturated fatty acids on cardiovascular risk factors: a systemic review and meta-analysis', *Ann Nutr Metab* 2011; 59: 176–86 doi: 10.1159/000334071.

78 Deutsche Gesellschaft für Ernährung DGE: Pressemitteilung aktuell 7. 2010, ‚Mehrfach ungesättigte Fettsäuren senken das Risiko für koronare Herzkrankheiten', http:/www.dge.de/uploads/media/DGE-Pressemitteilung-aktuell-07–2010-SFA-PUFA.pdf).

79 Joint FAO/WHO Expert Consultation on Fats and Fatty Acids in Human Nutrition, November 10–14, 2008, Geneva (2010), 'Interim summary of conclusions on dietary recommendations on total fat and fatty acids', (http://dx.doi.org/10.1159 %2F000331214).

80 Haudigorametto, F. et al., 'Study on the thermal stability of APA and DHA in Mujahir (Oreochromis Mossambicus) Fish Oil', Chemistry Department Faculty of Mathematics and Natural Sciences, Gjadialh Madla University Yogiakartza. Indonesia Indonesian J of Chemistry vol 5(2) ISSN 1411 3421.

81 Pak, C. S. et al., 'Stability and quality of fish oil during typical domestic application', Fishering Training Program, Sonsan Univerity of Fisheries, Kangwon Province, D.P.R, of Korea, Final project 2005.

82 Brenna, J.T. et al., 'Alpha linoleic acid supplementation and conversion to N-3 long-chain polyunsaturated fatty acids in humans', volume 80, Nr. 2–3, 2009 Feb–Mar 85–91 ISSN 0952–3278.

83 Gerster, H., 'Can adults adequately convert alpha-linoleic acid (18/3 N3)', *Int J Vitam Nutr Res*, 1998; 68(3), 159–73. PMID: 9637947.

84 Lands, W. E. M., 'Fish Omega 3 and human health', American Oil Chemists Society, 2005, ISBN 978–1-893997-81-3.

85 Simopoulos A.P.: *The importance of the ration of omega-6/omega 3 essential fatty acids*. Biomedicine & Pharmacotherapy 56(8) 365–97 PMID: 12442909.

86 Simopoulos, A.P., 'Importance of the Ratio of Omega-6 / Omega-2 Essential Fatty Acids: Evolutionary Aspects', and Simopoulos A.P. et al., 'Omega 6/Omega-3 Essential Fatty Acids Ratio: The Scientific Evidence', *World Review of Nutrition and Dietetics*, 92 pp 1–22 ISBN 3–8055-7640-4, PMID: 1457 9680, 2003.

87 Campbell, T.M., *The China Study: the most comprehensive Study of Nutrition ever conducted and the startling Implications for Diet, Weight loss and Long-term Health*, Perseus Distribution, June 2006, ISBN 978-1-932100-66-2, S. 444.

88 Sijbrands, E.J. et al., 'Mortality over two Centuries in large pedigree with familial hypercholesteraemia: family tree mortality study', *BMJ* 2001 Apr 28; 322(7293) 1019–23.

89 *BMJ* 991 oct.12: 'Risk of fatal coronary heart disease in familial hypercholestererolemia', 303(6807), 803–06.

90 Sijbrands, E.J. et al., 'Mortality over two Centuries in large pedigree with familial hypercholesterolaemia: family-tree mortality study', *BMJ* 2001 Apr 28; 322(7293) 1019–23.

91 Zapeta, R. et al., 'Gallbladder mortality and lithogenesis in obese patients during diet-induced weight loss', *Dig-Dis-Sci* 2000 Feb, vol. 45(2), 421–28, ISSN 0163–2116.

92 Tandon, R.K. et al., 'Dietary habits of gallstone patients in Northern India', *J. Clin Gastroenterology* 1996 Jan, vol: 22(1) 23–27, ISSN 0016–0790

93 Thomas, L.A. et al., 'Mechanism for the transit-induced increase in colonic deoxycholic acid formation in cholesterol cholelithiasis', *Gastroenterology* 2000 Sep.vol: 119(3) 806–15, ISSN: 0016–5085.

94 Bircher-Benner, Maximilian, *Ordnungsgesetze des Lebens*, Edition Bircher-Benner, Braunwald, 2014, S. 63, ISBN 378–3-906089-01-0.

95 'Pfizer gets sued over Celebrex', 27 Feb 2006, (http://money.cnn.com/2006/02/27/news/companies/celebrex/).

96 Hil, Vorwurf der Cholesterinlüge entkräftet' (http//www.aerzteblatt.de/v4/archiv/artikel.asp), *Deutsches Ärzteblatt*. Jg 36, Nr. 105, 2008, S. 1812.

97 NHLBI: 'ATP Cholesterin Guidelines' (http//:www.nhlbi.nih.gov/guidelines/cholesterol//) 18.11.2008.

98 Krmholz, H.M. et al., 'Lack of Association between Cholesterol and Coronary Heart Disease Morality and Morbidity and All-Cause Mortality in Persons older than 70 years', *JAMA* 1994; 272(17) 1335–40.

99 Ulmer, H. et al., 'Eve is not Adam: prospective follow-up in 149,650 women and men of cholesterol and other risk-factors related to cardiovascular

and all-cause mortality', *Journal of women's health* 2002 band 13(1) 2004 Jan–Feb S. 42–53, ISSN 1540–9996.
100 Gebbers, J.E. et al., 'Cholesterin ist für die Arteriosklerose ohne Bedeutung: die Ergebisse der Autopsien stützen die Lipidhypothese nicht', *Ars Medici* 1998; 88564–69.
101 Editorial, 'Central Nervous System and Limb Anomalies in case reports of first trimester Statin exposure', *New E J Med* 2004 Apr 8; 350(15) 1579–82.
102 'White Moms with low Cholesterol levels preemies more', *Los Angeles Times,* 1 Oct 2007.
103 Editorial, 'Cognitive impairment associated with atorvastatin and simvastatin', *Pharmacotherapy,* 2003 Dec 23(12) 1663–67.
104 Arzneimittelkommission der Deutschen Ärzteschaft, Akuter Gedächtnisverlust unter Atorvastatin und Simvastatin', (UAW-News International) (http://www.akdae.de/Arzneimittelsicherheit/Bekanntgaben(Archiv/2005/797_20050204.html), Feb 2005, downloaded 26 Feb 2014.
105 Prospective Studies Collaboration, 'Cholesterol, diastolic blood pressure, and stroke: 13,000 strokes in 450,000 people in 45 prospective cohorts', *Lancet* 1995(346) 1647–53.
106 Emond, M.J., 'Prognostic value of Cholesterol in Women of different ages', *J. Woman Health* 1997(6) 295–307.
107 Colomb B.A. et al.: *Statins lower blood pressure: results from the UCSD Statin-Study.* Circulation 2004(110, Suppl III) III-402 (abstract 1904.
108 Edward, C. et al., 'Relations of Trait Depression and Anxiety to low Lipid and Lipoptrotein Concentrations in healthy young adult Women', Pschosomatic Medicine 1999(61) 273–79.
109 Steffens, D.C., 'Cholesterol lowering Medication and relapse of Depression', *Psychopharmacol Bull* 2003; 73(4) 92–98.
110 Knashawn, M. et al., 'Simvastatin Causes Changes in Affective Processes in Elderly Volunteers', *J of the Am Geriatr Society*, Vol 54 P.70 Dec 2006.
111 Agargun, M.Y. et al., 'Nightmares and Serum Cholesterol Level: A primary report', *The Can J of Psychiatr,* May 2005.
112 Smak, P.H.G., 'Atorvastatin may cause nightmares', *BMJ* 2006, 332, S. 950.
113 Mikus, C.R. et al., 'Simvastatin impairs exercise training adaptations', *J of the Am College of Cardiology*, April 2013 ISSN 1558–3597.
114 MED-Watch-Meldung zur IMNM, 'HMG Co-A-Reductase Inhibitor (statin) drug-risk of immune-mediated necrotizing myopathie (IMNM) Label Changes', (http://www.fda.gov/Safety/MedWatch/Safety Information/ucm327852.htm), Oct 2012.
115 Mucchiano, G. et al., 'Age-related Amyloid in the Aorta', *Amyloid and Amyloidosis*, Springer Link, p. 402–404, 1990.
116 Cornwell III, G.G. et al., 'Senile cardiac Amyloidosis: demonstration of a unique fibril protein in tissue sections', *J Immnol.* 120: 1385–88.
117 Batttaglia S. et al.: *Aortenamyloidose im Erwachsenenalter.* Virchows Arch A Path Anat and Histol. 378; 153–159.
118 Muckle, T.J., 'Perpheral Angiopathy', *Amyloidosis*, Martinius Nijhoff Publishers, Dordrecht, 271–282.
119 Jenkins, D.J. et al., 'Glycemic Index: overview of implications in health and disease', *Am J Clin Nutr* 2002(76) 266–273.
120 Salmeron, J. et al., 'Dietary fiber, glycaemic load, and risk of non-insulin-dependent diabetes mellitus in women', *JAMA* 1997 (277), 472–77.
121 Salmeron, J., 'Dietary fiber, glycemic load, and risk of NIDDM in men', *Care* 1997, 20545–50.
122 Liu, S. et al., 'A prospective study of dietary glycaemic load and risk of myocardial infarction in women', *Am J Clin Nutr* 2000, 711455–61.
123 Jeppesen, J. et al., 'Effect of low-fat, high carbohydrate diets on risk factors for ischemic heart disease in postmenopausal women', *Am J Clin Nutr* 1997, 651027–33.
124 Liu, S. et al., 'A prospective study of dietary fiber intake and risk of cardiovascular disease among women', *Am J Coll Cardiol* 2002, 39 49–56.
125 Rimm, E.B. et al., 'Vegetable, fruit and dietary fiber intake and risk of coronary heart disease among men', *JAMA* 1996, 275447–451.
126 Pietinen, P. et al., 'Intake of dietary fiber and coronary heart disease in a cohort of Finnish men: the Alpha tocopherol, Beta-Caroten Cancer Prevention Study', *Circulation* 1996, 942720–2727.
127 Wolk, A.A. et al., 'Long term intake of dietary fiber and decreased risk of coronary heart disease among women', *JAMA* 1999; 2811998–2004.
128 Jacobs, D.R. et al., 'Fiber from whole grains, but

not refined grains, is inversely associated with all-cause mortality in older women: the JOWA women's-health study', *J Am Coll Nutr* 2000; 19(3 suppl) 236S-33=p.

129 Rimm, E. et al., 'Folate and Vitamin B6 from diet and supplements in related risk of coronary heart disease among women', *JAMA* 1998, 279359–65.

130 Voutilainen, S. et al., 'Low dietary folate intake is associated with an excess incidence of acute coronary heart events: the Koupio Ischemic Heart Disease risk Factor Study', *Circulation* 2001, 1032674–80.

131 Bazzano, L. A. et al., 'Dietary intake of folate and risk of stroke in US men and women', NHANES-I Epidemiologic Follow-up Study, *Stroke* 2002, 331183–89.

132 Lora, C. M. et al., 'Serum folate and cardiovascular disease mortality among US men and women', *Arch Intern Med* 2000, 1603258–82.

133 Voutilainen, S. et al., 'Low serum folate concentrations are associated with an excess incidence of acute coronary events: the Kuopio Ischemic Heart Disease Risk Factor Study', *Eur J Clin Nutr* 2000, 54424–28.

134 Vermeulen, E. G. et al., 'Effect of homocysteine-lowering treatment with folic acid plus vitamin B6 on progression of subclinical atherosclerosis: a randomized placebo-controlled trial', *Lancet* 2000, 355517–522.

135 Schnyder, G. et al., 'Decreased rate of coronary restenosis after lowering of plasma homocysteine levels', *N Engl J Med* 2001, 3451593–600.

136 Bostom, A. G. et al., 'Power shortage: clinical trials testing the "homocystein-hypothesis" against a background of folic acid-fortified cereal grain flour', *Ann Int Med.* 2001, 135133.37.

137 Kris-Etherton, P. M. et al., 'The effects of nuts on coronary heart disease', *Nutr Rev* 2001, 59103–11.

138 Hu, F. B. et al., 'Frequent nut consumption and risk of coronary heart disease: prospective cohort study', *BMJ* 1998, 3171341–1345.

139 Brown, L. et al., 'Nut consumption and risk of coronary heart disease in patients with myocardial infarction', *FASEB* J 1999, 13 A4332.

140 Ellsworth, J. L. et al., 'Frequent nut intake and risk of death from coronary heart disease and all causes in postmenopausal women: the Iowa Women's Health Study', *Nutr Metab Cardiovasc Dis.* 2001, 11372–77.

141 Albert, C. M. et al., 'Nut consumption and decreased risk of sudden cardiac death in the physicians health study', *Arch Intern Med* 2002, 1621382–87.

142 Kris-Etherton, P. M. et al., 'The effects of nuts on coronary heart disease risk', *Nutr Rev* 2001, 59103–111.

143 Mölgard, J. et al., 'Alfalfa seeds lower low-density lipoprotein, cholesterol and apolipoprotein B concentrations in patients with type II hyperlipoproteinemia', *Atherosclerosis* 651987 173–9.

144 Watzel, B. et al., *Bioaktive Substanzen in Lebensmitteln*, Hippokrates-Verlag, Stuttgart ISBN 3–7773-1115-4 1995.

145 Beecher, G. R. et al., 'Analysis of micronutrients in foods', Moon, T. E. and Micozzi, M. S. (eds), *Nutrition and cancer prevention: Investigating the roles of micronutrients*, Decker, New York, 1988, p. 103–58.

146 Apiz-Castro, R. et al., 'The anti-platelet principle of garlic, synergistically potentiates the antiaggregatory action of prostacyclin, forskolin, indomethacin and dipiridamole on human platelets', *Thromb Res* 421986 303–11.

147 Hertog, M. G. E. et al., 'Dietary oxidant flavonoids and risk of coronary heart disease: the Zutphen elderly study', *Lancet* 3421993 b 1997–2011.

148 Knekt, P. et al., 'Antioxidant vitamin intake and coronary mortality in a longitudinal population study', *Am J Epidemiol.* 1994, 1391180–89.

149 Knekt, P. et al., 'Antioxidant vitamin intake and coronary mortality in a longitudinal population study', *Am J Epidemiol* 1004: 1391180–89.

150 Gillman, M. W. et al., 'Protective effect of fruits and vegetables on development of stroke in men', *JAMA* 1995, 2731113–1117.

151 Gaziano, J. M. et al., 'A prospective study of consumption of carotenoids in fruits and vegetables and decreased cardiovascular mortality in the elderly', *Ann Epidemiol* 1995, 5 255–60.

152 Joshipura, K. J. et al., 'Fruit and vegetable intake in relation to risk of ischemic stroke', *JAMA* 1999, 2821233–39.

153 Joshipura, K. J., 'The effect of fruit and vegetable intake on risk for coronary heart disease', *Ann Intern Med* 2001, 1341106–14.

154 Liu, S. et al., 'Fruit and vegetable intake and risk of cardiocascular disease: the Women's Health Study', *Am J Clin Nutr* 2000, 72922–928.

155 Liu, S. et al., 'Intake of vegetables rich in carotenoids and risk of coronary heart disease in men: the Physicians' Health Study', *Int J Epidemiol* 2001, 30130–35.

156 Bazzano, L.A. et al., 'Fruit and vegetable intake and risk of cardiovascular disease in US adults: the first National Health and Nutrition Examination Survey Epidemiologic follow-up Study', *Am J Clin Nutr* 2002, 76 93–99.

157 Jacobs, D.R. et al., 'Whole grain intake may reduce the risk of ischemic heart disease death in postmenopausal women: the Iowa Women's Health Study', *Am J Clin Nutr* 1998, 68248–57.

158 Liu, S. et al., 'Whole grain consumption and risk of coronary heart disease: results from the Nurses' Health Study', Am J Clin Nutr 1999, 70412–19.

159 Liu, S. et al., 'Whole grain consumption and risk of ischemic stroke in women: a prospective study', *JAMA* 2000: 2841534–40.

160 Ornish D. et al., 'Can lifestyle changes reverse coronary heart disease? *The Lifestyle Heart Trial*' (see comments), *Lancet* 1990 Jul 21, vol 336(8708) pp. 129–33, ISSN 0023–7507.

161 Shai, I et al., 'Dietary intervention to reverse carotid atherosclerosis', *Circulation* 2010 Mar 16, 121(10): 1200–1208.

162 Rauma, A.L. et al., 'Vitamin B-12 status of long-term adherents of a strict uncooked vecan diet ("living food diet") is compromised', *Journal of Nutrition* Oct 1995(125) 2511–5.

163 Donaldson, M.S., 'Metabolic vitamin B-12 status on a mostly raw vegan diet with follow-up using tablets, nutritional yeast, or probiotic supplements', *Annuals of Nutrition and Metabolism* 2000: vol 44, pp. 229–34.

164 Sever, P.S. et al., 'Blood pressure and its correlates in urban and tribal Africa', *Lancet* 2 (1980), 60–64.

165 Andersen, J.W. et al., 'Plant fiber and blood pressure', *Ann internal Med* 98 (1983), 842–46.

166 Tesfaye, F. et al., 'Association between body mass index and blood pressure across three populations in Africa and Asia', *J of Human Hypertension* 207(21) 28–37.

167 Brown, W.J. et al., 'The Australian Longitudinal Study of Women's Heath', *Bulletin on the World Health Organisation*, Nov 2007 85(11) 886–887.

168 Ley, R.A. et al., 'An obesity associated gut microbiome with increased capacity for energy harvest', Nature 2006 Dec 21444(7122): 1027–31.

169 Backhed, F. et al., 'Mechanisms underlying the resistance to diet-induced obesity in germ-free mice', *Proc Natl Acad Sci USA*, 2007 Jan 16, 104 (3): 979.84. Epub 2007 Jan 8.

170 Backhed, F. et al., 'The gut microbiota as an environmental factor that regulates fat storage', *Proc Natl Acad Sci USA*, 2004 Nov 2: 101(44): 15718–24, E pub 2004 Oct 25.

171 Brilla, C.G. et al., 'Mineralocorticoid excess, dietary sodium and myocardial fibrosis', *J of Laboratory and Clin Medicine* 1992, 120(6) 893–901.

172 Sacks, F.M. et al., 'Effects of blood pressure of reduced dietary sodium and dietary approaches to stop hypertension(DASH) diet', Dash sodium collaborative research group, *N Engl J Med* 2001 Jan 4: 344(1) 3–10.

173 Taylor, R.S. et al., 'Reduced dietary salt for the prevention of cardiocascular disease: a meta-analysis of randomized controlled trials (Cochraine review)', *Am J Hypertens* 2011 Aug 24(8) 843–53.

174 Berkow, C.E. et al., 'Blood pressure regulation and vegetarian diets', *Nutr Rev* 2005 Jan; 63(1): 1–8.

175 Yokoyama, Y. et al., 'Vegetarian diets and blood pressure: a meta-analysis', *YAMA Intern Med* 2014 Apr, 174(4) 577–87.

176 Sacks, F.M. et al., 'A dietary approach to prevent hypertension: a review of the Dietary Approaches to stop Hypertension (DASH) Study', *Clin Cardiol* 1999 Jul 22 (7 suppl) III 6–10.

177 Appel, L.J. et al., 'Dietary approaches to prevent and treat hypertension: a scientific statement from the American Heart Association', *Hypertension* 2006 Feb: 47(2) 296–308.

178 Most, M.M., 'Estimated phytochemical content of the dietary approaches to stop hypertension (DASH) diet is higher than in the Control Study Diet', *J Am Diet Assoc* 2004 Nov: 104(11): 1725–7.

179 Sacks, F.M. et al., 'Blood Pressure in Vegetarians', reprint requests to Dr. Kass, Harvard Medical School, 774 Albany Street, Boston Massachusetts 02118.

180 Oude Griep, L.M. et al., 'Processed fruit and vegetable consumption and 10-year stroke incidence in a population-based cohort study in the Netherlands', *Eur J Clin Clin Nutr* 2011: 65791–99.

181 John, J.H. et al., 'Effect of Fruit and vegetable consumption on plasma antioxidants concentrations on blood pressure: a randomized controlled trial', *Lancet* 2002, 3591969–1974.

182 Elliott, P. et al., 'Dietary phosphorus and blood pressure: international study of macro- and micro nutrients and blood pressure', *Hypertension* 2008, 51669–75.

183 Joffres, M.R. et al., 'Relationship of magnesium intake and other dietary factors to blood pressure: the Honolulu heart study', *Am J Clin Nutr* 1987, 45469–75.

184 Rock, C.L. et al., 'Bioavailability of beta-carotene is lower in raw than in processed carrots and spinach in women', *J Nutr* 1998: 128913–16.

185 Chan, Q. et al., 'Relation of raw and cooked vegetable consumption to blood pressure: the INTERMAP Study', *J of Human Hypertension* 2014 28, 353–9.

186 Jenkins, D.J.A. et al., 'Effect of a six month vegan low carbohydrate ("Eco Atkins") diet on cardiovascular risk factors and body weight in hyperlipidaemic adults: a randomized controlled trial', *BMJ* open 2014, 4, e003505, Google Schola CrossRed.

187 Fontana L. et al., *Long-term low caloric low protein vegan diet and endurance exercise are associated with low cardiometabolic risk,* Rejuvenation Res 2007 10225–234.

188 McEvoy, C.T. et al., 'Long term vegetarians have low oxidative stress, body fat and cholesterol levels', *Nutr Res Pract* 2012, 6, 155–61.

189 Nochols M. et al., *Trends in age-specific coronary heart disease mortality in the European Union over three decades: 1980–2009,*. European Heart J Bd 34, (39) Oct 2013 3017–27.

190 Colonna, P. et al., 'Nonpharmacologic care of heart failure: counseling, dietary restriction, rehabilitation, treatment of sleep apnea, and ultrafiltration', *Am J Cardiol* 2003, May 8, 91(9A) 41F-50F.

191 Rothberg, M.B. et al., 'The new heart failure diet: less salt restriction, more micronutrients', *J Gen Med* 2010 Oft 25(10) 1136–37.

192 Känig, G and Vancura, I., *Neue chinesische Akupunktur*, Verlag Wilhelm Maudrich, Wien, München, Bern, 1989.

193 Heine, H. et al., *Das System der Grundregulation* (48), Haut-Verlag, Heidelberg, 1990.

194 Hertog, M.G.L. et al., 'Dietary oxidant flavonoids and risk of coronary heart disease: The Zutphen eldery study', *Lancet*, 342 (1993 b) 1997–11.

195 Apiz-Castro, R. et al., 'The antiplatelet principle of garlic synergistically potentiates the anti-aggregatory action of prostacyclin, forskolin, indomethacin, dipyridamol on human platelets', *Thrombosis Research* 42 (1986) 303–11.

196 Andersen, J.W., 'Plant fibers and blood pressure', *Ann Internal Med* 98 (1983) 842–6.

197 Watzl, B. and Leitzmann, C., *Bioaktive Substanzen in Lebensmitteln*, Hippokrates-Verlag Stuttgart, ISBN 3-7773-1115-4, 1995.

Index

ACE inhibitors	51	Antiarrhythmics	76
Acetyl salicylic acid	57	Anticoagulation	63, 64, 65, 70, 76
Acetyl salicylic acid, aspirin	41, 94		
Acupuncture and TCM	84	Antioxidative substances and systems	21, 94
Acupuncture of the skull according to Yamamoto	70	Aorta	14
		Aortal valve	14
Adenosine	47, 77	Aortal valve stenosis	63
ADH (antidiuretic hormone)	48	Aortic insufficiency	64
Adiposity	19, 23, 49, 59, 95	Apoplexy, epidemiology	69, 72
		Apoplexy (stroke, cerebral infarction)	19, 63, 69, 72
Adrenaline	46, 52, 74		
Age and coronary heart disease	34	Apparent health	19
Ageing, premature	21	Arachidonic acid	28
AIDS	50, 80	Arrhythmia	57, 66, 74
Ajoene in garlic	41	Arrhythmia, absolute	75
Alcohol	19, 66, 75	Arteria carotis	14
Aldosterone	30, 48	Arteria hepatica	14
Alliin of Garlic and Onion	40, 47	Arteria lienalis	14
Alveolas	15	Arteria mesenterica	14
Alzheimer's disease	21, 37, 41	Arteria subclavia	14
Amaurosis fugax (temporary blindness)	72	Arterioles	14, 48
		Arterioles, sclerotisation	47
Amyloid, amyloidose	32, 37	Arteriosclerosis	11, 18, 21, 38, 40, 61, 62, 63, 71, 86
Amyloid, amyloidosis	21		
Amyotrophische lateralsklerose (ALS)	21		
		Arteriosclerosis, dietary reduction	25, 43, 88
Anaemia	59	Arteriosclerosis, epidemiology	19
ANCA antibodies	79	Arteritis	71, 80
Aneurysm	22, 68	Arteritis temporalis Norton (giant-cell arteritis, A. cranialis)	80
Aneurysma dissecans of the aorta	68		
Aneurysm of the cerebral arteries	68	Aschoff-Tamara-node (AV-node)	14, 74
Angina Pectoris	22, 54	Ascites	65
Angina pectoris, CSS-classification of severity	54	Aspergillus carditis	66
		Asthma bronchiale and fatty acids	28
Angina pectoris, epidemiology	55	AT1-antagonists (sartans)	51
Angina pectoris, homoeopathic therapy	54	Ataxia (gait disorder)	69
		Atrial fibrillation and stroke risk	75
Angina pectoris, stable	54	Atrial fibrillation causes	75
Angina pectoris, unstable	54	Atrial fibrillation, epidemiology	75
Angiotensin	48	Atrial fibrillation, intermittent	75
Anthocyanins, aubergines, blueberries	40	Atrial fibrillation, tachycard	75, 76

Atrial flutter and atrial fibrillation	61, 63, 69, 70, 75	Cardiac shock	57
Atrium tachycardia	77	Cardiomyopathy	62
Auricle, closing the	76	Cardioversion	76
Autoimmune diseases	28, 71, 79	Carotenoids	40, 41, 94
AV-nodal reentry, tachycardia	77	Carotid stenosis	72
AV-node (Aschoff-Tamara-node)	14, 74	Carotid vein congestion	65
AV-node, double formation	77	Catalase	21
		Catheter ablation	76
Balloon catheter dilatation	57, 63	Catheter dilatation	71
Baroreceptors	48	Cerebral haemorrhage (haemorrhagic infarction)	22
Basic regulation system	15, 16	Cerebral vasculitis	80
Basic substance of the soft connective tissue	15, 22, 37	CHA$_2$DS$_2$VASC-Score for indication of anticoagulation	76
Basic substance of the tender connective tissue	31	Chagas-disease	66
Behcet syndrome (vasculitis with arthritis)	80	Chemotherapy, damage to the heart	62, 66
Beta blockers	52, 76	Chlorophyll	16
Beta-cryptoxanthin	49	Cholesterol	23
Bile acid	30	Cholesterol breakdown	31
Bile acids, primary, secondary	40	Cholesterol breakdown, receptor path	43
Biochemistry	17	Cholesterol level	32, 39
Blood pressure amplitude, increased (between both values)	64	Cholesterol metabolism	30
Blood pressure centre	48	Cholesterol synthesis	31
Blood pressure regulation	48	Cholesterol transport	30, 31
Blood type A and heart-attack risk	57	Cholestyramin	34
Blood volume, regulation	48	Chorea Huntington	21
Bradycardia (too slow heart rhythm)	74	Chorea minor (Huntingdon's disease)	61
Breathlessness	64, 65	Chronic rheumatic heart disease	61
Buddenbrook syndrome	54	Chylomicrons	14, 31
Bundle branch block, 2		Citrate synthetase	36
1 block	77	CKMB	56
Burnout syndrome	46	Claudicatio intermittens (intermittent claudication)	22, 44, 73
Butter, cream	29	Climate therapy for cardiovascular patients	82
Butyric acid	26, 90	Clopidogrel	57
		Cocaine and vasculitis	80
Caffeine	47	Coenzyme Q 10	21
Calcium	52	Coffee	43, 88
Calcium antagonists	52, 77	Coherence	16, 17
Calorie calculation	16, 23	Coherence principle of Prigogine	17
Cancer	21, 28, 41	Competitive sports as a cause of atrial fibrillation	75
Capillaries	15	Complement	79
Capillary microscopy	15, 21	Complex carbohydrates	38
Capillary network of the intestinal mucosa	14	Conducting information	15
Carbohydrates and arteriosclerosis	38	COPD (chronic obstructive pulmonary disease)	50, 59
Cardiac insufficiency, biventricular	62, 63, 75	Coronary drug project	24

Coronary Primary Prevention Trial	23	Endotoxins of the intestine and hypertension	46
Coronary sclerosis	54, 74	Energy, orderly, chaotic	16
Coronary syndrome, acute	56	Enterohepatic cycle	23, 40, 95
Cortisol	30	Enteroviruses (carditis)	66
Coumarins (anticoagulation)	76	Environmental stress and heart-attack risk	57
Coxsackie viruses (carditis)	66	Eosinophil granulomatosis (Churg-Strauss syndrome)	79
Cryoglobuline vasculitis	79	EPA (eicosapentaenoic acid)	27
Cutaneous leucocytoclastic angiitis	80	Epidemiology of the cardiovascular diseases	11
Cytochrome P 450-Oxidase	20	Ergotamine arteritis	80
Danish Diet Cancer and Health Study	76	Erythema anulare	61
DASH-Study on hypertension	49	Essential fatty acids	26
Defibrillation	57, 78	Estradiol	30
Dental root abscesses, hypertension, Angina pectoris	46, 54	Excessive stress and hypertension	46
Depression and statins	36	Expansion receptors of the atria of the heart	48
DHA (decosahexaenoic acid)	27	Extractive substances in meat broth	46
Diabetes mellitus	18, 25, 27, 33, 39, 57, 59, 95	Extrasystoles (skipped heartbeats)	65, 75
Diabetic neuropathy	21	Extrasystoles, supraventricular	74
Diastole	14		
Dietary fibre, fibres, effect	39, 47, 94	FATS (familial atherosclerosis treatment study)	24
Difficulty in swallowing (dysphagia)	69	Fatty acids\ Ratio of omega 8 to omega 3 fatty acids, short-chained	47
Digitalis	60, 76	Fatty acids, types and importance	26
Diltiazem	76	Fatty liver	25
Diuresis (urination)	60	Fatty streaks	18, 32
Diuretics	51	Fearfulness and hypertension	46
Diuretics, herbal	51	Feeling of life	16
DNA-peroxidation	21	Fish oils	27
Dominance of the faster frequency	14	Flavonoids	41, 49
Double images (seeing double)	69	Flaxseed oil	28
Dromotropic effect	14	Flexibility of the Red Blood Cells	15, 23, 51, 90
Echo viruses (carditis)	66	Foam cells	18, 22, 32
Elaidic acid	29	Foleic acid, risk of heart attack and apoplexy	40
Electrocardiogram	56, 74	Framingham study	62
Electro conversion	76, 77	Free radicals	21
Electrolyte balance, disorder	74	French paradox	19
Electro smog	18, 43	Fresh food, vegetarian, importance	22
Embolism	76	Fresh raw fruit and vegetable food	17
Embolism of the brain	69		
Endangiitis obliterans, vasculitis from smoking	80	Gallstones	32
Endarterectomy (removal of the arteriosclerosis in layers)	72	Garlic	40, 41, 47
Endocarditis	61, 62, 63, 67	Gas exchange	15
Endocarditis prophylaxis	65		
Endocardium	13		
Endothelium	13		

GLAS (cholesterin-lowering atherosclerosis study)	24	Idiopathic lone atrial fibrillation	75
Glutathion	21	IgA antibodies	81
Glutathione reductase	21	IgA-vasculitis Schönlein-Henoch	79
Glycaemic index	38	IgG4-testing of food incompatibilities	81
Glycemic load	39	Immune system, and highly unsaturated fatty acids	28
Granulomatosis with polyangiitis Wegener	79	Immuno-competence	81
		Immunosuppressive therapy, carditis	66
Haemorrhagic brain infarction (cerebral haemorrhage)	22	IMNM (immune-mediated necrotizing myopathy)	36
HAS-BLED-Score for indication of anticoagulation	76	Inflammation processes and fatty acids	28
HDL cholesterol	95	Inflammatory diseases of the heart (carditis, endocarditis, myocarditis)	66
Healthful teas	131	Information	17
Heart attack	19, 56	Information of life	16
Heart attack, complications	57, 62	Inhibition of blood clotting	76
Heart attack, epidemiology	18, 56	Inhibition of blood clotting by plant food	41
Heart attack, risk factors	57	Inotropic effect	14
Heart attack, silent	56	Insulin	38
Heart attack, survival	57	Insulin resistance	39
Heart valve defects	61, 75	Insult and hypertension	46, 57
Heavy metals and hypertension	46	Interleukin	22
Heidelberg vegetarian study	24	INTERMAP Study	49
Helsinki Heart Study	23	Intermittent claudication (s. Claudicatio intermittens)	73
Hepatitis	79	Intestinal flora	23, 44, 46
HMG-CoA-reductase	31, 34	Intestinal symbiosis (impaired intestinal flora)	23
Holiday Heart Syndrome	75	Intima	21
Holter long-term ECG	70	Inuit and arteriosclerosis	45
Homocystein level	40		
Homoeopathic treatment	83	Juvenile, rheumatic polyarthritis	61
Human protein needs	37		
Hydrotherapy for cardiovascular patients	82	Kawasaki syndrome	80
Hypercholesterolemia	32	Lack of movement, movement training and arteriosclerosis	18, 34, 49
Hypertension	34, 45, 57, 75	Lack of sleep	43
Hypertension, dangerous risks	47	Lack of vital substances	43
Hypertension, epidemiology	49, 76	LASER-amplification of the UV light in the DNA	16
Hypertension, essential	46	LASER threshold	16, 17
Hypertension, malignant	71	LDL cholesterol	22
Hypertension, psychosomatic partial causes	46	LDL cholesterol, oxidation	33
Hypertension, pulmonary (lung hypertension)	50	LDL-receptor path	31
Hypertension, therapy with medication	51	Leakage radiation	16
Hyperthyrosis	74, 75	Lens cataract, cataract and diet	41
Hypertrophy, eccentric	64		
Hypertrophy of the heart muscle	47, 63, 65		

Leptin and regulation of body weight	48
Life energy	17
Life expectancy, improvement in cardiovascular diseases USA	10
Life information	17
Lip cyanosis	64
Lipoproteins LDL, VLDL, IDL	31
Liver cirrhosis	65
Loss of consciousness (syncopes)	50
Loss of field of vision	69
Low-cholesterol diet	33
Lucerne	40
Lung emphysema	50
Lung oedema	59, 63
Lutein	49
Lycopens	49
Lyme disease of the heart	66
Macrophages	18, 22, 35
Magnesium	43
Magnetic stimulation, transcranial	70
Malformations from statins	35
Managers' disease	46, 54
Margarines	29
Matrix	15
Memory loss, LDL cholesterol, statins	31, 35
Mesenterial infarction	22
Metabolism economy	43
Migraine	19, 57, 69
Minerals, importance, alkaline	43
Mitochondria	20, 36
Mitral insufficiency	62
Mitral valve	14
Mitral valve prolapse	62
Mitral valve stenosis	61
Morphine	57
Movement training and statins	36
MPA (microscopic polyarteritis PAN)	79
Multiple risk factor intervention trial	24
Multiple sclerosis	41
Mumps carditis	66
Muscle cramps	28
Muscle pain	36
Myocardial fibrosis	49
Myocardial infarction, posterior	56
Myocardial infarction, septal	56
Myocarditis	66
Myopathy, toxic, statins	36

Naturopathic blood-pressure-reducing medication	53
NCEP (National Cholesterol Education Program)	23
NECP III risk groups	33
Neglect	69
Neural therapy	70
Neural therapy of the heart's sympathetic nervous system	75, 77, 84
Neurohypophysis	48
Neurothrombectomy	70
Nightmares	36
Nitrites	65
Nitroglycerine	54, 57, 84
NOAC (new oral anticoagulants)	76
Nosocomial endocarditis (from resistant home and hospital germs)	67
NSTEMI (non ST-elevation myocardial infarction)	56
Obstipation and gallstones	32
Obstipation and hypertension	46
Omega-3 fatty acids	23, 26, 27
Omega-6 fatty acids	26, 27
Order therapy	11
Ornish-study, Ornish diet	24
Oxidation of the fatty acids and the LDL-Cholesterol	40, 43, 95
Oxidative stress	20
Pancarditis	66
Pancreatitis, chronic and alcohol	20
Parasympathetic nervous system	14, 74
Parvo virus (carditis)	66
PDV (peripheral vascular disease)	68, 73
Pectins	47
Pelvic artery	14
Pericapillary inflammation	22
Pericardium	13
Peroxide dismutase	21
Phosphates, energy-rich (ADP, ATP)	26, 38
Phosphatidylcholin	24
Photon storage	16
Photosynthesis	11, 16
Phytosterins	40, 49
Polyarteritis temporalis (PAN)	80
Polyphenols	41
Portal vein system	14, 31
Positive dromotropic effect	14

Positive inotropic effect	14	Risk factors for coronary heart disease	34
Posterior myocardial infarction	56, 62	Risk factors of the arteriosclerosis	18, 20, 63
Potassium	43	Risk of haemorrhage and anticoagulation	76
Potential of the cell membrane	47	Roasted substances	11
Pregnancy and statin risk	35	Roasting byproducts	46
Pregnenolone	30	Roasting substances	43
Prinzmetal's angina	54, 56	Rolling up	15
Progesterone	30	R.O.S. (reactive oxygen species)	21
Prostaglandine and fatty acids	28		
Protein economy	37	Saponins	40
Protein peroxidase	21	Sarcoidose	50
Proteins and arteriosclerosis	37	Scavenger pathway	32
Proteoglycans	15	Schönlein-Henoch Purpura	79
PTA (percutaneous transluminal angioplasty)	71	Sclerodermia	50
Pulmonary circulation	15	Secondary arteritises	80
Pulmonary embolism	65	Secondary plant substances (phytochemicals)	21, 39, 41
Pulmonary hypertension	50, 62, 64	Selenium	21
Pulmonary valve	13, 15	Sense of life, life against one's own	46
Pulmonary valve insufficiency	64	Sickle-cell anaemia	50
Pulmonary valve stenosis	64	Sinus node	14
Pulmonary vein isolation	77	Sinus rhythm	74
Pulmonary vein stenosis	77	Sinus tachycardia	77
Pulse deficit (pulse slower than heartbeat)	77	Skipped heartbeats (extrasystoles)	65, 74
Pump capacity of the heart	13	Sleep	13, 14
Purkinje fibres	14	Sleep apnoea syndrome	60
		Smoking	18, 20, 34, 50, 80
Racing heart (s. tachycardia)	65, 77	Sodium/potassium gradient	47
Radiation, damage to the heart from	62	Sodium/potassium pumps	47
Raw-food studies on hypertension	49	Specific dynamic effect	37
Raw-food studies, protective effect against arteriosclerosis	41	Statin medication, problem and side effects	34
Raw food, vegetarian, importance	52	STEMI (ST-elevation myocardial infarction)	56
Raynaud's phenomenon	50	STENT	57
Reducing cholesterol, medication, statins	34	Still's disease	61
Regeneration	16	Stimulants	11
Rejection crises after transplantation and vasculitis	80	Storage of information	15
Renal artery stenosis	71	Streptokinase	57
Renal insufficiency (renal failure)	59, 63	Stress	18, 43
Renin	48, 71	Stroke (apoplexy)	19, 69
Reserpine	53	Stroke, cerebral infarction	19
Rhabdomyolysis, fatal side effect of statins	36	Stroke unit	70
Rheumatic fever	61, 62, 63, 65	Subarachnoid haemorrhage	19, 69
Rheumatoid arthritis and fatty acids	28	Sugar and arteriosclerosis	38
Rhythm amplitude at atrial fibrillation	76	Superfine flours and arteriosclerosis	39
		Sympathetic nervous system	14, 74

Syncopes (loss of awareness)	53, 76	Vaccenyl-docosahexoaenyl acid	24
Syncopes (loss of consciousness)	50	Valve replacement	62
Syphilis arteritis	80	Valvuloplasty	62
Systemic circulation	14	Valvulotomy	65
Systole	14	Vasculitides, treatment	80
		Vasculitis	72, 79
Table salt	43, 45, 49, 51	Vaso vasorum	22
Tachycardia, paroxysmal	77	Veganism	31
Tachycardia (racing heart)	65, 74, 77	Vegetarianism	31
Takayasu arteritis	80	Vegetarian studies	49
TAVI (transcatheter aortic-valve implantation)	64	Venous congestion, acute	65
		Ventricular fibrillation	57, 66, 75, 78
Terrain treatment for cardiovascular patients	82	Verapamil	76
		Viscosity of the blood	23
Theophylline	47	Vitamin A	21
Thrombocyte aggregation inhibition	69	Vitamin B 6	40
Thrombolysis therapy	57	Vitamin B 12	44
Thrombosis	28, 71	Vitamin C	21, 40
Thromboxan	41	Vitamin D	19, 30, 57
Thromboxane	94	Vitamin E	21, 40
TIA (transient ischaemic attack)	69		
Tocotrienols of the whole-grain	40	Weight reduction	60
Toxic myocardial damage	66	Whole-grain and heart attack risk	39, 40
Trans-fatty acids	29	Wolff-Parkinson White syndrome	77
Tricuspid valve	13, 15		
Tricuspid valve insufficiency	65	Xanthines, importance	41
Tricuspid valve stenosis	65		
Triglycerides	24, 39	Zeaxanthin	49
Troponin	56		
Trypanosoma carditis	66		
Two to One Relation (2:1)	23		

CENTRE FOR SCIENTIFIC NATURAL MEDICINE

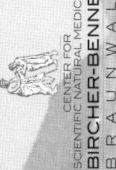

SCIENTIFIC NATURAL MEDICINE
BIRCHER-BENNER
B R A U N W A L D

People come to the Bircher-Benner Medical Centre from a large number of countries in search of healing.

Here, you will be valued as a unique person, listened to and understood. Here, humanity and dignity are important and the medicine is a noble undertaking.

The search for the true causes of diseases is central to our work, as is the inclusion of your self-curative powers in the process of healing.

Centre for scientific natural medicine

Our fresh-vegetable diet will bring about a rapid change in your metabolism; natural regulative therapies take precedence where possible.

The atmosphere and the living tradition of the Bircher-Benner Centre, where novelty and modernity are combined with decades of experience, contribute to your healing.

The doctors and therapists will treat you personally and have all the facilities of a modern clinic at hand when needed.

The supplementation of traditional medicine by the regulative diagnosis and therapy of natural healing often permits a cure where the usual therapies have failed.

In the Medical Centre, you can relax and recover, and will experience the deep regeneration of your healing powers.

CENTRE BIRCHER-BENNER
CH-8784 Braunwald

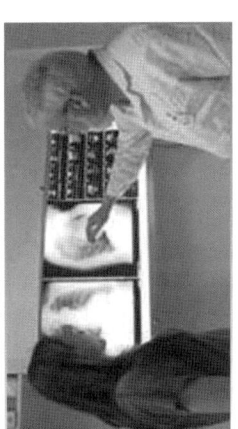

Phone: +41 (0)21 801 60 04
Fax: +41 (0)55 643 16 93
info@bircher-benner.com
www.bircher-benner.com

Indications: any internal diseases, migraine, tinnitus, neuralgia and other pain conditions, fibromyalgia, arthritis and arthrosis, collagenoses, liver, gallbladder and gastrointestinal diseases, metabolic diseases and diabetes, cardiovascular diseases, kidney and prostate diseases, women's diseases, allergies, skin diseases, convalescence, fatigue, depression and anxiety, menopausal, hormonal and weight problems.